Symptom Control

in Advanced Cancer

Roger Woodruff

with an Introduction by

Michael H. Levy, MD, PhD

Asperula Pty Ltd
Melbourne

USA Edition

National Library of Australia Cataloguing-in-Publication Data

Woodruff, Roger
Symptom Control in Advanced Cancer

Bibliography
Includes index
ISBN 0646331922
1. Cancer pain - Treatment. 2 Cancer - Palliative treatment.   I. Title

Published by   Asperula Pty Ltd
                      Suite 9, 210 Burgundy Street
                      Heidelberg, 3084
                      Victoria, Australia

Printed in Australia by Australian Print Group, Maryborough, Victoria

NOTICE

Whilst every effort has been made to ensure that the patient care recommendations in this book, including the indications and dosages for drug therapies, are correct and in keeping with accepted standards of practice at the time of publication, neither the author nor the publisher can accept any legal responsibility or liability for any errors or omissions that may be made.

It is the responsibility of the reader, before using any drug, to consult the manufacturer's product information sheet in order to check recommended doses, warnings and contraindications. This is particularly important with new or infrequently used drugs.

Table of Contents

Good symptom control is fundamental to the opportunity
to care for the whole person.

Jo Hockley[1]

Meticulous attention to detail can lead to
appropriate and effective treatment to the end of a patient's life.
This transforms his experience, and the memories of his family.

Dame Cicely Saunders[2]

1. Hockley J. Rehabilitation in palliative care. *Palliative Medicine* 1993; 7 (suppl 1) : 9-15
2. Saunders C in Twycross RG and Lack SA. *Therapeutics in Terminal Cancer*. Churchill Livingstone, 1990

Introduction

There is a new groundswell of interest in end-of-life care in the USA spawned by the growing demands for cost reduction by managed care, recurring requests for physician assisted suicide by fearful consumers, and the disappointing documentation of inadequate terminal care by the SUPPORT study. Organized and academic medicine are finally addressing what this country's hospice movement has been practising and promoting for over twenty three years. More exciting than the realization that dying patients need better palliative care is the recognition that patients should not wait until their last few months of life to receive appropriate relief of their symptoms and attention to their psychological and spiritual needs. Effective palliative care must be offered early in conjunction with disease-oriented, curative, life-prolonging therapies. Once such therapies are deemed no longer effective, appropriate, or desired, palliative care assumes priority in the form of interdisciplinary hospice care to optimize quality of life and quality of death.

Cancer accounts for sixty percent of the patients cared for by the over 2,000 hospice programs in this country. One in two cancer deaths were cared for by US hospice programs in 1996. At the core of interdisciplinary hospice care is superb medical care focused upon effective control of physical symptoms. Successful palliation of symptoms throughout the cancer trajectory helps patients cope with their cancer and its therapy. Palliative care is an active therapeutic option that must be learned by all health care professionals and offered to all cancer patients.

This book provides a concise, systematic approach to the palliation of common symptoms experienced by patients with advanced cancer. For each symptom, Dr. Woodruff delineates potential causes, typical clinical features, appropriate assessment, diagnosis specific therapy, and general symptomatic treatment. He stresses the importance of open communication with patients and families and respect for their autonomy in decision making and treatment planning. Treatment goals must be clear and diagnostic and therapeutic interventions must be appropriate to each patient's disease and prognosis. Each chapter has a section focusing upon the special concerns that arise when patients are in their final days of life. Dr. Woodruff's recommendations are universal and can be easily applied to patients and families in the USA.

Effective control of physical symptoms is the very least that should be promised to patients with advanced cancer. This book is an excellent resource for all clinicians charged with this clinical mandate, physicians and nurses, oncologists and family physicians. Symptom control opens the door to the relief of psychosocial and spiritual distress. Such comprehensive, palliative care reduces patient suffering and optimizes the quantity and quality of their lives. This book is a testament that there is never nothing more that can be done for patients with advanced cancer. There is always something that can be done. That something is competent, compassionate, palliative care.

Michael H. Levy, MD, PhD
Director, Supportive Oncology Program
     Fox Chase Cancer Center
     Philadelphia, PA
President-Elect,
     American Academy of Hospice and Palliative Medicine

Abbreviations

The following abbreviations are used in the text

routes of administration

IM	intramuscular
IV	intravenous
PO	oral
PR	rectal
SC	subcutaneous
SL	sublingual
TD	transdermal
ED	extradural
SA	subarachnoid

measures

μg	microgram
mg	milligram
g	gram
kg	kilogram
ml	millilitre
Gy	Gray, a measure of irradiation

preparations

cap	capsule
inj	injection
mixt	mixture
supp	suppository
tab	tablet
IR	immediate-release
CR	controlled-release
SR	sustained-release
EC	enteric-coated

frequency of administration

PRN	(*pro re nata*) as required
q	(*quantum*) frequency e.g. q4h is every 4 hours

procedures

ECG – electrocardiography
EMG – electromyography
CT scanning – computerised tomography
MRI scanning – magnetic resonance imaging

1 Symptom control in advanced cancer

Good symptom control is essential in the care of all patients with cancer, but it becomes even more important as the cancer progresses. At this stage, as the focus shifts from quantity to quality of life, effective symptom control is crucial. Skilful palliation of symptoms will not only improve physical comfort and quality of life, it will allow matters of psychosocial and spiritual suffering to be addressed, something which is not possible if patients have unrelieved pain or physical distress.

Causes

Knowledge of the various causes and pathophysiological processes which produce clinical symptoms is necessary for appropriate treatment decisions to be made. Many symptoms suffered by patients with advanced cancer have a number of possible causes and in some cases there are multiple causes in effect. In each situation, careful assessment is required to determine which cause (or causes) is responsible for a particular problem.

Assessment

Clinical assessment, with a careful history and examination, will often indicate the cause of a particular problem. In other situations, investigations may be required. Investigations should be employed if the results will influence treatment decisions and the treatment will improve, or at least maintain, the patient's quality of life. Investigations, particularly those involving invasive procedures, should be appropriate to the stage of the patient's disease and the prognosis.

Treatment

The principles of symptom control are listed in Table 1.1.

Table 1.1 Principles of symptom palliation

careful clinical assessment ± investigation
    caring manner
    continued commitment
good communication with the patient and family
    cause(s) of symptoms
    treatment options, including side effects
    goals of therapy
treatment
    appropriate to cause(s)
    individualized for each patient
    changed promptly if ineffective
    involve colleagues for difficult clinical problems
    consistent, not changed unnecessarily
    continued reassessment
    appropriate to the stage of the disease and prognosis
integrated into a comprehensive plan of multidisciplinary palliative care

A careful clinical assessment, with or without investigations, is made to determine the cause (or causes) of the patient's symptoms. This needs to be done in a caring way and requires continued commitment if the clinical problems respond poorly to initial therapy.

Good communication with the patient and family is important if symptom palliation is to be successful. They are informed about the cause of the symptoms and what treatment options are available. Both the benefits and possible side effects of any proposed treatment are discussed. The goals of therapy also need to be clear and patients receiving purely symptomatic treatment should know that it will have no effect on the underlying cancer.

The treatment given for the control of symptoms is determined by the cause or causes and depends on careful assessment. Treatment needs to be individualized and tailored for each patient and, given that many patients with advanced cancer are both elderly and frail, there may be considerable variation in the doses of medications required. Perseverance may be needed and if the first treatment employed is not successful, alternatives should be tried. Difficult symptom problems should be discussed with colleagues and no patient should ever be told "there is nothing more that can be done". Treatment should be consistent and not variable: if a particular medication is working satisfactorily it should not be changed unless there are sound medical reasons to do so. Whatever therapy is prescribed, a process of continued reassessment is important to assess the results of treatment and because modifications are frequently required as cancer progresses.

Treatment needs to be appropriate to the stage of the patient's disease and prognosis, as indicated in the tables of treatment options in this book. In most instances, therapy for a patient who is bed-bound or in the last days or week of life is quite different from what might be prescribed for a patient with a longer prognosis. The final paragraph in many sections in this book, labelled **Terminal care**, addresses what therapy is appropriate for patients in the terminal phase.

Effective symptom control is of fundamental importance but is only one aspect of care. Matters of psychological, social, cultural and spiritual suffering must also be addressed, although it is frequently necessary to first control pain and physical symptoms for this to be achieved. Symptom control, with the best possible medical and nursing care which is available and appropriate, should be an integrated part of a comprehensive and multidisciplinary approach to palliative care.

2 Respiratory

> dyspnea
> cough
> hemoptysis
> pneumonia
> pneumonitis
>
> pulmonary embolism
> pleural effusion
> hoarseness
> terminal respiratory congestion
> lung metastases

DYSPNEA

Dyspnea is breathlessness or an unpleasant sensation of difficulty breathing. Dyspnea is subjective and is always associated with some degree of anxiety, which in turn makes the dyspnea worse.

Cause (Table 2.1). Many patients have multiple causes; in others there may be no specific cause other than general debility.

Assessment. A clinical history and examination, together with knowledge about pre-existing lung disease, are often sufficient to determine the cause of dyspnea. A chest x-ray may show infiltration by primary or secondary cancer, with or without collapse distal to bronchial obstruction, or confirm the presence of a pleural or

Table 2.1   Causes of dyspnea

airway obstruction
    tracheal
        tumor of larynx, thyroid, mediastinum or bronchus
        tracheo-esophageal fistula
    bronchial
        tumor : intrinsic obstruction or external compression
        chronic bronchitis
        acute infection, bronchitis
        bronchospasm : bronchitis, asthma, carcinoid syndrome
reduction in functional lung tissue
    surgical resection : lobectomy, pneumonectomy
    tumor : atelectasis, lymphangitis, multiple metastases
    fibrosis : pre-existing, radiation, chemotherapy
    pleural effusion
    pneumothorax
    infection
    hemorrhage
    pulmonary embolism
    chronic emphysema
impaired ventilatory movement
    chest wall weakness, motor impairment, general debility
    chest wall pain
    elevated diaphragm : ascites, hepatomegaly, phrenic nerve lesion
cardiovascular
    congestive cardiac failure, cardiomyopathy
    pericardial effusion, constrictive pericarditis
    shock, hemorrhage, septicemia
anemia
anxiety

pericardial effusion. Lymphangitis carcinomatosis produces reticular markings radiating from the hilar region. The changes of radiation pneumonitis conform to the radiation field. Widespread or miliary markings are more difficult to interpret and can be due to multiple metastases, infection, hemorrhage or drug toxicity. Further tests including spirometry, arterial gases, ventilation-perfusion scanning, echocardiography and CT scanning should be considered if the results will significantly affect treatment decisions.

Treatment

Treatment of specific causes (Table 2.2). Treatment is directed at the underlying cause (Table 2.1) where possible. Dyspnea due to multiple metastases, lymphangitis carcinomatosis and radiation pneumonitis may improve with prednisolone 40-60 mg/d or dexamethasone 8-12 mg/d; the dose is weaned to the minimum effective dose after a few days. Nonmalignant causes of dyspnea, including chronic lung disease, bronchial asthma, heart failure and anemia are treated by standard means.

Table 2.2   Dyspnea : treatment options for specific causes

obstruction	endoscopic laser resection
	stenting
	external radiotherapy
	endoscopic radiotherapy (brachytherapy)
	corticosteroids
	systemic therapy (sensitive tumors)
	esophageal tube (for tracheo-esophageal fistula)
effusions	drainage
	instillation of sclerosants
	systemic therapy (sensitive tumors)
metastases	
solitary	surgery, corticosteroids, radiotherapy, systemic therapy (sensitive tumors)
multiple	corticosteroids, systemic therapy (sensitive tumors)
lymphangitis	corticosteroids, systemic therapy (sensitive tumors)
pneumonitis	
radiation	corticosteroids
chemotherapy	corticosteroids, stop chemotherapy
pneumonia	antimicrobial therapy
pulmonary emboli	anticoagulation
hemorrhage	treatment of systemic bleeding diathesis

> *Treatment must be appropriate to the stage of the patient's disease and the prognosis*

General symptomatic measures (Table 2.3). The dyspneic patient is managed in a calm and reassuring manner, given gentle and sure explanation about the dyspnea, and reassured that it can be treated and will not necessarily get worse. Pain, if present, should be adequately treated. Patients should be allowed to choose the position in which they are most comfortable, even if this means sleeping in a chair. Dyspneic patients frequently appreciate fresh cool air from a fan or open window. Breathing education and relaxation exercises will help control exacerbations of dyspnea and the associated anxiety. Patients with chronic dyspnea benefit from counselling regarding activity management and energy conservation techniques. Distraction therapy and massage help some patients.

Oxygen. Oxygen therapy is of benefit in patients with documented hypoxia (arterial p_aO_2 <60 mmHg or saturation <90%). If dyspnea occurs only intermittently or

Table 2.3 Dyspnea : general symptomatic measures

calm, reassuring attitude	aid expectoration
nurse patient in position of least discomfort	steam, nebulized saline
improved air circulation	mucolytic agents
distraction therapy	expectorants
relaxation exercises	physiotherapy
breathing control techniques	reduce excess secretions
counselling	anticholinergics
oxygen	antitussives

on exertion, patients should be encouraged to reserve oxygen therapy for exacerbations and before exercise. Oxygen therapy must be used with caution in patients with chronic obstructive lung disease who may have hypercapnia and depend on hypoxia for their respiratory drive. A portable oxygen concentrator is the easiest and most economic means of providing oxygen therapy at home.

Bronchodilators. These drugs are useful when there is a reversible element to bronchial obstruction. In the non-acute situation, the usefulness of these drugs should be documented by measuring peak flows before and after treatment. Bronchodilators in use include β-adrenergic stimulants (e.g. albuterol), anticholinergics (e.g. ipratropium) and the xanthine derivatives, aminophylline and theophylline (Table 2.4). The side effects of albuterol include tremor, tachycardia and headache. Xanthines may cause cardiac and cerebral stimulation and a number of drug interactions are documented.

Corticosteroids. Corticosteroids are effective bronchodilators and may also improve dyspnea associated with pulmonary metastases and lymphangitis carcinomatosis. In palliative care it is customary to start with a larger dose so as not to miss a therapeutic effect and then wean to the minimum effective dose after a few days.

Table 2.4 Dyspnea : examples of drug therapy*

bronchodilators
    albuterol by metered aerosol or 2.5-5 mg by nebulizer, q4-6h
    ipratropium by metered aerosol or 250-500 µg by nebulizer, q6h
    aminophylline, theophylline PO
corticosteroids
    prednisolone 40-60 mg/d PO, dexamethasone 8-12 mg/d PO
opioids
    morphine 5-10 mg PO, q4h or 4-hourly PRN
    morphine 5-10 mg by nebulizer, q4h or 4-hourly PRN
nebulized local anesthetics
    lidocaine 2%, 2.5-5 ml by nebulizer, q6h PRN
anxiolytics
    diazepam 2 mg PO q8h ± 5-10 mg nocte
    lorazepam 0.5-1 mg SL, q6-8h
mucolytics (for sputum retention)
    humidified air (steam, nebulized saline)
    acetylcysteine 10%, 6-10 ml by nebulizer, q6-8h
anticholinergics (for excessive secretions)
    scopolamine hydrobromide 0.4-0.8 mg IM q4h; 0.8-2.4 mg/d SC infusion
antitussives

* Nebulizer therapy for patients with chronic obstructive lung disease who
  may have hypercapnia should be with air, not oxygen.

Opioids. Morphine and other opioid drugs are the most useful agents in the treatment of dyspnea. In patients with cancer, morphine improves dyspnea without causing any significant reduction in various measures of ventilatory function. Care should be taken with patients with significant chronic lung disease but morphine-induced respiratory depression is rarely a clinical concern with medication given orally or by nebulizer. The recommended dose of morphine is 5-10 mg PO, 4-hourly, and titrated against effect and toxicity. Patients already receiving morphine for analgesia should have the dose increased by 25-50%.

Nebulized morphine. Nebulized morphine is effective for some patients with dyspnea including those already receiving systemic opioids for analgesia. Advantages of nebulized therapy include rapid effect and the possibility of fewer systemic side effects. The usual dose is 5-10 mg in normal saline, nebulized with air or oxygen, given 4-hourly or as required for dyspnea, and titrated against effect. A small proportion of patients will develop bronchospasm and the initial dose should be given in a situation where appropriate therapy is immediately available.

Nebulized local anesthetics. Nebulized local anesthetic agents help some patients with dyspnea and cough (see Cough).

Anxiolytics. Benzodiazepines may reduce dyspnea, probably by an anxiolytic and sedative effect. They are scheduled according to need: regularly through the 24 hours, only at night, or to counteract anxiety attacks.

Other drugs. Dyspnea aggravated by sputum retention or tenacious sputum can be helped by breathing humidified air (steam, nebulized saline) or by mucolytic agents such as acetylcysteine. Anticholinergic drugs are of benefit when excessive secretions contribute to dyspnea. Antitussives should be used if dyspnea is exacerbated by coughing.

Terminal care. In the last week or days of life, treatment should be purely symptomatic. Investigations have little place except for the patient who would be made more comfortable by the drainage of a significant pleural effusion. Antibiotic therapy is usually not warranted and may only serve to prolong the dying process. If of benefit, bronchodilator therapy can be continued by mask. Semiconscious or unconscious patients who still appear dyspneic should be treated with subcutaneous morphine.

COUGH

Cough is the physiological reflex employed to clear irritant, foreign or particulate material from the respiratory tract.

Cause. Cough can be caused by physical or chemical stimulation of receptors in both the upper and lower respiratory tract and also in the pleura, pericardium and diaphragm (Table 2.5).

Assessment. The clinical history, physical examination and chest x-ray will usually define the cause of cough. Bronchoscopy may be required to document endobronchial tumor.

Treatment

Treatment of specific causes. Where possible and appropriate, treatment should be directed at the underlying cause as described in the section on Dyspnea (Table 2.2). Cough caused by a post-nasal drip may improve with antihistamine or anticholinergic medication.

Table 2.5 Causes of cough

airway irritation
    atmosphere : smoke, fumes, dry atmosphere
    tumor : endobronchial tumor, extrinsic bronchial compression
    aspiration : vocal cord paralysis, reduced gag reflex, tracheo-esophageal fistula
    gastroesophageal reflux
    infection : post-nasal drip, laryngitis, tracheitis, bronchitis
    increased bronchial reactivity : ACE inhibitors, asthma
    sputum retention
    excess sputum (bronchorrhea)
lung pathology
    infection
    infiltration : primary or secondary cancer, lymphangitis carcinomatosis
    pneumonitis : radiation, chemotherapy
    chronic obstructive lung disease
    pulmonary fibrosis
    pulmonary edema : congestive heart failure, pericardial effusion with tamponade
irritation of other structures associated with the cough reflex
    pleura, pericardium, diaphragm

General symptomatic measures (Table 2.6). Atmospheric irritants should be avoided and smoking discouraged. Atmospheric humidification or humidification of the inspired air can be of significant symptomatic benefit.

Patients with a productive cough may benefit from measures which aid expectoration although this is not indicated for the terminally ill and may be distressing for patients who are weak and debilitated. Steam or nebulized saline are probably as

Table 2.6 Symptomatic treatment of cough

general measures	avoid smoke, fumes
	atmospheric humidification
	nurse patient in position of least discomfort
aid expectoration	
humidification	atmospheric humidification
	avoid dehydration
	humidified, nebulized air
mucolytics	steam or nebulized saline
	inhalations, e.g. menthol, eucalyptus
	chemical mucolytics, e.g. acetylcysteine
expectorants	e.g. ammonium chloride, iodides
drainage	physiotherapy, postural drainage
bronchodilators	if bronchospasm present
antibiotics	if infection present
reduce secretions	anticholinergics, opioids, antihistamines
antitussives	
opioids	codeine 8-30 mg PO q4h
	dihydrocodeine 10-15 mg PO q4-6h
	morphine 5-20 mg PO q4h
opioid analogues	dextromethorphan syrup 15-30 mg PO q4-6h
local anesthetics	lidocaine 2%, 2.5-5 ml by nebulizer, q6h PRN
sedation	benzodiazepines
	tranquillizers

effective as other mucolytic agents. Chemical expectorants are of questionable extra value and may cause nausea. Anticholinergic or opioid drugs are used for patients with excessive respiratory secretions.

Patients with a persistent dry cough are treated with antitussives. Corticosteroids may be of benefit by their effect on bronchial compression or lymphangitis carcinomatosis. Pharyngeal irritation can be treated with simple linctus or a proprietary cough syrup.

Opioids. The antitussive drugs in clinical use are opioids or opioid analogues and act by central suppression of the cough reflex. The opioid drugs are superior antitussives but cause more sedation and constipation. Meperidine is not antitussive. The dose and timing of antitussive medication is tailored to suit the individual patient and may only be required at night.

Nebulized local anesthetics. Local anesthetics, administered by nebulizer, may be of benefit in the treatment of intractable cough. A small proportion of patients will develop bronchospasm and the first dose must be given in a situation where appropriate therapy is immediately available. Other side effects include pharyngeal numbness and loss of the gag reflex; patients should be offered a drink immediately before treatment and then fasted for 1 to 2 hours.

Cough related to tracheo-esophageal fistula. Patients with tracheo- or broncho-esophageal fistulas complain of paroxysmal coughing immediately after swallowing. These fistulas will not close spontaneously, even if effective radiotherapy or systemic therapy is given. Dietary manipulations are usually unsuccessful and feeding by a nasogastric tube or gastrostomy is often necessary. Some patients obtain good relief with the endoscopic placement of a well-fitting esophageal tube.

Terminal care. Treatment is with an opioid drug which will also act to dry respiratory secretions. Antibiotics and vigorous physical therapy are inappropriate. Sedatives may be of benefit at night and haloperidol, which will dry respiratory secretions by its anticholinergic effect, is preferable to a benzodiazepine. Smoking can be discouraged but, as the respiratory benefits of stopping smoking may take a month to be manifest, forcing terminally ill patients to stop smoking may compound their misery.

HEMOPTYSIS

Cause (Table 2.7).

Table 2.7 Causes of hemoptysis

tumor	primary, metastatic
infection	bronchitis, pneumonia
pneumonitis	radiation, chemotherapy
pulmonary embolism	
cardiac failure	
bleeding diathesis	thrombocytopenia, coagulopathy
trauma	endotracheal tube, bronchoscopy

Assessment. Hemoptysis should be distinguished from gastrointestinal and nasopharyngeal bleeding: hemoptysis is associated with coughing, the blood is usually bright and frothy and often mixed with phlegm. The cause of hemoptysis is usually apparent from the clinical history and examination. A chest x-ray may provide further information.

Treatment

Hemoptysis frequently provokes considerable anxiety. The fear is that massive hemorrhage may follow smaller hemoptyses but, as this occurs rarely, the patient and family should be reassured.

Treatment of tumor-related hemoptysis depends on the severity (Table 2.8). Radiotherapy is effective for the majority of patients but may require bronchoscopy for treatment planning. Hemoptysis not directly related to tumor is treated appropriately.

Table 2.8 Treatment options for hemoptysis related to tumor

mild	reassure
	tranexamic acid 1g PO q8h
	corticosteroids
moderate or persistent	radiotherapy
	endobronchial radiotherapy (brachytherapy)
	laser coagulation
massive	morphine

Massive hemoptysis. Massive hemoptysis, due to infiltration of a pulmonary artery, is rare. It is a terminal event and the patient rapidly becomes unconscious as a result of hypoxia and hemorrhage. There is a brief period during which patients may experience suffocation, during which time they should never be left unattended. If possible, they are treated promptly with morphine by injection to allay anxiety and fear. If a massive hemoptysis is anticipated, diazepam and morphine should be readily available, as well as colored towels or blankets to cover or mask the blood.

Terminal care. Hemoptysis occurring in terminally ill patients should be managed with reassurance and explanation, to both patient and family. Antitussives may reduce the amount of hemoptysis. Antibiotics are usually inappropriate.

PNEUMONIA

Treatment

The management of pneumonia in patients with advanced cancer must be appropriate to the stage of the disease and the prognosis. Intensive treatment is only appropriate if it is felt that successful treatment of the chest infection will allow the patient to survive a significant period of time with reasonable quality of life.

Localized infection which may be secondary to bronchial obstruction by tumor is treated with appropriate antimicrobial therapy and treatment to relieve the bronchial obstruction (radiotherapy or endobronchial laser therapy). Physiotherapy and postural drainage are important.

Pneumonia presenting as a diffuse infiltrate has to be distinguished from drug-induced pneumonitis, miliary metastases and lymphangitis carcinomatosis. If clinically appropriate, treatment is with intravenous broad spectrum antibiotics, modified according to response and the results of cultures. If there is continued lack of improvement, open lung biopsy may be the only means to establish the diagnosis and exclude miliary metastases or drug induced pneumonitis. For patients with a shorter life expectancy, intensive therapy with intravenous antibiotics may be inappropriate and oral antibiotics should be considered.

Terminal care. In the last days or week of life, antibiotic therapy is usually inappropriate and is seldom effective. Dyspnea, cough, pain and fever are treated symptomatically.

PNEUMONITIS

Radiation pneumonitis

Acute. The incidence and severity of acute radiation pneumonitis depend on treatment factors including the volume irradiated and the dose given. It usually develops within a few weeks of treatment. Patients complain of dyspnea and nonproductive cough which vary from mild to distressing. There are crepitations and rales in the affected area and there may be a pleural friction rub. Chest x-ray shows hazy shadowing or 'ground glass' opacification in the treated area, with margins conforming to the treatment field. If causing significant symptoms, treatment is with prednisolone 50-100 mg/d, continued for several weeks. The dose is then cautiously reduced over a number of weeks, the rate being determined by the patient's symptoms.

Chronic. Acute pneumonitis may progress to chronic fibrosis over a period of 6 months to 2 years. The fibrosis causes dyspnea which may be mild or severe. Chest x-ray shows fibrotic scarring with shrinkage of the lung in the treated area. Treatment is symptomatic.

Chemotherapy-related pneumonitis

Some chemotherapy drugs can cause pneumonitis and the onset may be delayed for several months after the offending drug has been stopped. Drug induced pneumonitis causes dyspnea and a nonproductive cough. The clinical features range from a mild and transient illness to rapidly fatal respiratory failure. Examination reveals crepitations and rales and the chest x-ray shows a diffuse reticular/nodular pattern. The differentiation of drug toxicity from infection or malignant infiltration is difficult and may require consideration of a lung biopsy.

Treatment. The offending drug or any suspected drug is stopped. Corticosteroids in moderate dosage, prednisolone 40-100 mg/day, are helpful in some cases. Treatment is otherwise symptomatic.

PULMONARY EMBOLISM

Clinical features. The clinical manifestations depend on the size and number of emboli and the general condition and cardiorespiratory reserve of the patient. Major pulmonary emboli cause acute dyspnea, pleuritic pain, hemoptysis and an infiltrate on chest x-ray; large or multiple emboli may cause acute cardiovascular collapse and sudden death. Alternatively, a small embolus may cause only transient dyspnea and tachypnea without other signs. Multiple small emboli may cause progressive dyspnea without pain, hemoptysis or chest x-ray signs and are only diagnosed by a lung scan.

Assessment. The diagnosis of pulmonary embolism may be clinically obvious and can be confirmed with a ventilation perfusion scan. A scan is indicated if active therapy is contemplated and in those patients with otherwise unexplained progressive dyspnea.

Treatment

The treatment of pulmonary embolism in patients with advanced cancer requires careful consideration of the potential benefits and complications. Standard therapy with heparinization for 5 to 10 days, followed by oral anticoagulation for three months or more, is appropriate for patients whose prognosis is several months or more. Patients with a shorter life expectancy may benefit from initial heparinization, which often helps resolve the acute dyspnea and pleuritic pain, although subsequent oral anticoagulation with its attendant risks may be considered unwarranted. Patients with recurrent pulmonary emboli, and those for whom anticoagulation is difficult or contraindicated, may be considered for the insertion of a vena caval Greenfield filter. Thrombolytic therapy is usually considered to be contraindicated in patients with cancer (see Thrombosis, Chapter 6).

Terminal care. Pulmonary embolism is a not uncommon terminal event and is managed by symptomatic treatment of pain and dyspnea.

PLEURAL EFFUSION

Clinical features. Pleural effusions cause dyspnea, a nonproductive cough, pleuritic pain and characteristic physical signs. Chest x-ray will confirm the presence of an effusion which is usually unilateral in the case of malignant infiltration.

Assessment. Simple pleural aspiration with biochemical and cytological examination (Table 2.9) will usually document the cause of an effusion. Malignant cells are seen in 50-80% of effusions due to pleural infiltration by tumor. CT scanning will provide more detail regarding underlying pathology and the presence of mediastinal disease in patients with a chylous effusion. Thoracoscopy, with visualization of the pleura and direct biopsy of suspicious lesions, should be considered if doubt exists as to the cause of an effusion.

Table 2.9   Pleural effusion : etiology and fluid characteristics

	Transudate / Exudate	*Cytology*
inflammation of pleural surface		
infiltration by tumor	E	+*
infection, infarction, irradiation	E	-
lymphatic obstruction		
peripheral obstruction by tumor	T or E	+/-†
central (mediastinal) obstruction	E (chylous)	-
raised pulmonary venous pressure		
local venous obstruction by tumor	T or E	+/-†
cardiac failure, pericardial tamponade	T	-
other edematous conditions		
hypoproteinemia, renal failure, liver failure	T	-

* positive fluid cytology depends on whether tumor cells are shed into the fluid
† positive fluid cytology depends on there being pleural infiltration by tumor in addition to blockage of the veins or lymphatics

Treatment

There are a number of different approaches to the management of pleural effusions (Table 2.10). Selection depends on clinical circumstances and particularly on the patient's condition and prognosis. Patients with small or asymptomatic effusions require no therapy.

	Advantages	*Disadvantages*
repeated pleural aspiration	simple procedure	repeated procedures cumulative protein loss increased risk of infection, pneumothorax, fluid loculation
pleural aspiration and instillation of sclerosant	simple procedure	fluid drainage may be suboptimal lung expansion cannot be checked more risk of loculation
tube drainage and instillation of sclerosant (± thoracoscopy)	allows complete drainage lung expansion checked tube causes pleuritis and aids pleurodesis less risk of loculation	(minor) surgical procedure longer hospital stay

thoracotomy and pleurodesis or pleurectomy	highly effective	major surgical procedure
		   for tube pleurodesis failures or if
		   thoracotomy indicated for
		   other reasons

Table 2.10   Pleural effusion : therapeutic alternatives

> *Treatment must be appropriate to the stage of the patient's disease and the prognosis*

Repeated aspiration. Repeated pleural aspiration is suitable if only a limited number of procedures are likely, as with patients whose effusions reaccumulate only very slowly, the terminally ill and those responding to systemic therapy.

Pleurodesis. Pleurodesis involves the instillation of a sclerosant substance to obliterate the pleural space and prevent reaccumulation. Pleurodesis is best performed after complete drainage of the pleural fluid using an intercostal catheter or at the time of thoracoscopy. Video-assisted thoracoscopy is a relatively minor procedure and is suitable for many patients with advanced cancer. Patients too weak for a drainage procedure should be treated by aspiration alone as their prognosis does not warrant attempted pleurodesis.

Tetracycline has in the past been the sclerosant of choice but is no longer available. Talc is an excellent sclerosing agent and is suitable for use at the time of thoracoscopy. Talc should not be used if there is pleural infection. Fever and pain are frequent side effects of talc instillation and the solution should be mixed with local anesthetic before injection.

Thoracotomy. Thoracotomy with talc poudrage or pleurectomy are highly effective in preventing recurrent pleural effusions but should be reserved for effusions which have recurred despite tube drainage and pleurodesis or if thoracotomy is performed for other indications.

Pleuro-peritoneal drainage. A pleuro-peritoneal catheter can be used for troublesome effusions in patients who are not considered suitable for other procedures because of age, general frailty or poor prognosis. The catheter is placed in the subcutaneous tissue and has a valved chamber which allows fluid to be manually pumped against the normal pleuro-peritoneal pressure gradient.

Chylous effusions. Chylous effusions are caused by disruption of the thoracic duct and treatment is usually by radiotherapy to the mediastinum. Repeated pleural aspiration is ineffective and attempts at pleurodesis are unsuccessful.

Terminal care. Pleural aspiration in the terminally ill should only be considered if it is felt drainage will produce significant symptomatic benefit. For most patients, symptomatic treatment of dyspnea, pain and cough is all that is required.

HOARSENESS

Cause. Hoarseness may be caused by local laryngeal pathology or damage to the vagus nerve, particularly the recurrent laryngeal branch (Table 2.11).

Table 2.11 Hoarseness

laryngeal disease	*recurrent laryngeal nerve*
infection	surgery to neck, thorax
voice abuse	cancer : intracerebral, neck, thorax
harsh coughing	infection : herpes zoster
radiotherapy	
endotracheal intubation	
bronchoscopy	

Clinical features. Recurrent laryngeal nerve palsy causes hoarseness and the characteristic ineffectual 'bovine' cough. Because of the inability to close the cords, the explosive element of the cough required to clear secretions is lost or diminished.

Assessment. Laryngoscopy will demonstrate laryngeal disease or, with laryngeal nerve palsy, paralysis of the cord on one side. Clinical examination usually allows localization of a neurological cause: intracranial pathology will be associated with other cranial nerve lesions as well as cerebellar and long tract signs; lesions at the base of the skull cause abnormalities of the IXth, Xth, XIth cranial nerves together (jugular foramen syndrome); lesions lower in the neck and in the thorax cause only laryngeal signs and, in the absence of a palpable mass or recent surgery to the neck, the lesion is likely to be in the mediastinum.

Treatment

Laryngeal disease is treated appropriately. If feasible, nerve lesions causing vocal cord paralysis are treated with radiotherapy. Patients with troublesome symptoms due to vocal cord paralysis may be treated by injection of teflon into the affected cord. This improves both the voice and the quality of the cough, but requires a general anesthetic.

TERMINAL RESPIRATORY CONGESTION

Terminal respiratory congestion or 'death rattle' is the rattling, noisy or gurgling respiration caused by the accumulation of pharyngeal secretions in patients who are unconscious, semiconscious or too weak to expectorate.

Treatment

Patients should be positioned on their side and this may be all that is required. Oropharyngeal suction should be reserved for unconscious patients, as it may be more distressing to the patient than their gurgling breathing.

Anticholinergic drugs are used to suppress the production of secretions (Table 2.12). Scopolamine hydrobromide may be given as repeated subcutaneous injections or as a continuous infusion. Scopolamine hydrobromide may cause sedation and occasionally produces paradoxical excitation. Atropine may cause bradycardia after repeated injections. Transdermal scopolamine patches have the benefit of being effective for 72 hours, but the onset of action is delayed for several hours and other anticholinergic treatment is needed during this period.

Table 2.12	Treatment of terminal respiratory congestion
injection	scopolamine hydrobromide 0.4 mg SC q2-4h *or* 0.6-1.2 mg/24h SC infusion
	atropine 0.6 mg SC q2-4h
transdermal	scopolamine hydrobromide 1.5 mg patch q72h

LUNG METASTASES

Clinical features (Table 2.13). Pulmonary metastases are often asymptomatic. Growth of the metastases may lead to extrinsic bronchial compression or involvement of the pleura or pericardium. Chest wall invasion is less common than with primary lung cancer. Involvement of hilar nodes may produce lymphangitis carcinomatosis. Secondary metastases to the mediastinal nodes may cause compression of various structures (Table 2.13). Endobronchial metastases occur infrequently and hemoptysis is less common than with primary tumors.

Table 2.13	Symptoms and signs of lung metastases
metastases to lung parenchyma	asymptomatic
	dyspnea
	extrinsic bronchial compression
	cough
	wheeze and stridor
	segmental or lobar collapse
	predisposition to infection
pleural infiltration	pain, pleural effusion
cardiac involvement	pericardial effusion
mediastinal involvement	tracheal obstruction
	esophageal obstruction
	superior vena caval obstruction
	lymphatic obstruction
	lymphangitis carcinomatosis
	chylous pleural effusion
	recurrent laryngeal nerve palsy
	phrenic nerve palsy
endobronchial metastases	cough, hemoptysis

Treatment

Anticancer therapy. Patients with sensitive tumors should have a trial of systemic therapy. Radiotherapy is of benefit for hemoptysis or pain secondary to infiltration and can be considered for a large metastasis causing symptoms. Surgery is not indicated in patients with advanced cancer.

Symptomatic measures. Treatment is otherwise symptomatic, as outlined in the other sections in this chapter. Patients with widespread metastases or lymphangitis carcinomatosis may benefit from corticosteroids (prednisolone 40-60 mg/d) although the effect may last only a few weeks.

Further Reading - see page 111

3 Gastrointestinal

xerostomia	fecal incontinence,
stomatitis	rectal discharge
alteration of taste	perianal and vulval pruritus
nausea and vomiting	flatulence
hiccups	stomas
dysphagia	fistulas
esophagitis	lower gastrointestinal bleeding
upper gastrointestinal bleeding	ascites
indigestion	liver metastases
bowel obstruction	hepatic failure and
constipation	encephalopathy
diarrhea	biliary tract obstruction

XEROSTOMIA (DRY MOUTH)

Xerostomia is dryness of the mouth.
Cause (Table 3.1).

Treatment

The treatment of xerostomia includes avoidance of any causative or aggravating factors, attention to oral hygiene and various means of stimulating salivary flow (Table 3.2). The patient's drug therapy should be reviewed. Commercially available mouth washes that contain alcohol are avoided as they may have a drying effect. Dietary salivary stimulants may be helpful. Pharmacological sialogogues (e.g. bethanechol 10 mg q8h) help some patients but are contraindicated in patients with bowel or urinary obstruction or asthma; others feel that side effects (sweating, flushing, urinary frequency, intestinal colic) outweigh any benefit. Commercially available salivary substitutes can be used before meals and at bedtime. Patients with severe xerostomia are advised to use a fluoride toothpaste as well as fluoride brush-on gels and rinses.

Table 3.1 Causes of xerostomia

decreased production of saliva	extensive mucosal damage
dehydration	erosion
salivary gland disorder	infiltration
radiotherapy	infection
radical surgery	radiotherapy
malignant infiltration	neutropenic mucositis
sialadenitis	increased evaporation
infective, obstructive	mouth breathing
xerostomia of age	hyperventilation
anxiety	smoking
drugs	dry atmosphere
diuretics, anticholinergics, opioids	oxygen therapy
tranquillizers, antidepressants, antihistamines	

Table 3.2 Treatment of xerostomia

treat or avoid causative or aggravating factors
    drugs, dehydration, dry atmosphere, smoking, anxiety
oral hygiene
    mouth washing, lip care, dental hygiene, denture care
topical therapy to prevent infection
frequent fluids
dietary advice
    soft moist foods, appetizing, nutritionally adequate
stimulation of saliva
    dietary   sucking ice cubes, frozen tonic water, citrus drinks, pineapple,
                    ascorbic acid lozenges, sugarless gum, slowly dissolving sweets
    sialogogues   bethanechol, neostigmine, pilocarpine
artificial saliva
fluoride gels and rinses

Terminal care. Mouth care is important during the terminal phase. Keeping the oral mucosa moist and clean will relieve discomfort, prevent stomatitis and reduce any sensation of thirst caused by dehydration. This can be achieved by regular mouth washes and the use of sprays or atomizers.

STOMATITIS

Stomatitis is inflammation, infection or ulceration of the mouth.
Cause (Table 3.3).

Table 3.3 Stomatitis : causative and predisposing factors

chemotherapy	direct mucosal damage, neutropenic mucositis
radiotherapy	direct mucosal damage, xerostomia
xerostomia	diminished amount of less alkaline saliva
poor oral hygiene	gingivitis, dental caries, poorly fitting dentures
malnutrition	thin atrophic mucous membranes
infection	fungal, viral, bacterial, aphthous ulcers
drugs	steroids, antibiotics predispose to fungal infection

Clinical features. The main symptom is pain. If severe, it may prevent eating or drinking and cause difficulty taking analgesics and other medications.

Treatment

Preventive. All patients with advanced cancer, particularly those receiving chemotherapy or radiotherapy, require a program of regular mouth care to prevent stomatitis (Table 3.4). Prophylactic antifungal therapy should be considered for all patients at risk of stomatitis and the addition of an antiseptic reduces the incidence of bacterial stomatitis in myelosuppressed patients.

Table 3.4 Preventive mouth care

observation	regular program of daily inspection
regular washing	saline or commercial mouthwash (avoid mouthwashes with alcohol)
	antifungal therapy
	antiseptic (e.g. chlorhexidine, povidone-iodine) if myelosuppressed
lip care	petroleum jelly
dental hygiene	regular brushing with soft brush
denture care	dentures cleaned after each meal, stored overnight in weak antiseptic
dietary advice	avoidance of very hot or very hard food

Treatment of pain. Mild to moderate pain can usually be managed using mouthwashes containing anesthetic or analgesic agents, with or without oral analgesics (Table 3.5). Severe pain is treated with opioid analgesics; parenteral morphine is used if necessary.

Table 3.5   Stomatitis : analgesic and anesthetic preparations

local anesthetics	
lidocaine	viscous 2% : 15 ml q4h, rinse and expel
cocaine	solution 0.5% : 10 ml q4h, rinse and expel
non-steroidal anti-inflammatory drug	
benzydamine	solution 0.15% : 15 ml q4h, rinse and expel
salicylate	
choline salicylate	gel - apply with gentle massage q4-6h
mucosal protective agent	
sucralfate (1 g tab dissolved in 10 ml)	mouthwash q4h

Active treatment. The mainstay of therapy is regular mouth washing to clean away debris and to keep the mucous membranes moist. Mouthwashes containing alcohol or phenol should be avoided as they may cause pain and further damage. The cheapest is a saline mouthwash made by adding a teaspoon of salt to a liter of water. If there is encrusted debris, sodium perborate is effective; an alternative is a saline and soda solution made by adding one teaspoon each of salt and sodium bicarbonate to a liter of water.

Treatment of infection. Specific antimicrobial therapy is given if the causative organism is known. If it is uncertain, mouthwashing with povidone-iodine solution is recommended, as it has activity against bacteria, fungi and viruses.

Candidiasis. Candidiasis is treated topically for 7 to 10 days (Table 3.6). In severe cases, ketoconazole given for 5 days is effective but may be hepatotoxic. Fluconazole is an alternative which is not hepatotoxic but is more expensive. Severely immunosuppressed patients may require continuing topical therapy or weekly oral fluconazole prophylaxis.

Table 3.6   Stomatitis : treatment of fungal infection

nystatin	suspension	100,000 U/ml	1 ml q4-6h
	lozenge	100,000 U	q4-6h
ketoconazole	tablet	200 mg	once daily x 5d
fluconazole	tablet	150 mg	once daily x 5d

Bacterial infection. Antibiotics for bacterial stomatitis are selected on the basis of culture results but should cover gram negative organisms.

Viral infection. Herpes labialis is treated with topical aciclovir ointment and is most effective if used frequently during the prodrome (Table 3.7). Herpetic gingivostomatitis is treated with povidone-iodine mouthwash and aciclovir.

Table 3.7   Stomatitis : herpetic infection

labialis	aciclovir 5% cream
	povidone-iodine 10% paint or ointment
gingivostomatitis	povidone-iodine 7.5%, diluted 1:20
	aciclovir : 200 mg, five times daily, PO or IV, for 7-10 days

Aphthous ulceration. Aphthous ulceration is treated with topical tetracycline (tetracycline suspension 250 mg, as a mouthwash, 6-hourly) or corticosteroid (triamcinolone 1% in orabase, applied topically, 6-hourly).

Terminal care. Continued mouth care is important in maintaining comfort. Severe pain should be managed with parenteral opioid analgesics. Topical antimicrobial therapy can be continued if it is causing no distress and it is considered that it may help control pain.

ALTERATION OF TASTE

Taste may be reduced (hypogeusia), lost (ageusia) or distorted (dysgeusia). **Cause** (Table 3.8).

Table 3.8 Causes of altered taste

reduced number of taste buds
surgery, radiotherapy, chemotherapy, old age
impaired taste bud cell renewal
chemotherapy, radiotherapy, poor nutritional state
impaired taste bud stimulation
poor oral hygiene, necrotic tumor, stomatitis, xerostomia
cranial nerve and brain stem lesions
drugs
chemotherapy, drugs causing xerostomia
metabolic disturbances
hypopituitarism, hypoadrenalism, diabetes, renal failure
cancer *per se*

Treatment

Management (Table 3.9) includes treatment of the cause, care in the preparation and presentation of food, and the use of appetite stimulants (see Anorexia, Chapter 12).

Table 3.9 Management of alteration of taste

treatment of cause	mouth care : general oral hygiene, stomatitis, xerostomia
	neurological lesions
	metabolic disorders
	drugs
presentation of food	discuss choice with patient and dietician
	food : hot, strong aromas, strong and tart tastes
	visually appealing
	avoid noxious smells
appetite stimulants	corticosteroids, alcohol, progestogens

NAUSEA AND VOMITING

Nausea is the unpleasant subjective feeling of the need to vomit. Retching consists of rhythmic spasmodic contractions of the diaphragm and abdominal muscles. Vomiting is the expulsion of the gastric contents through the mouth caused by forceful contraction of the abdominal muscles and diaphragm.

Physiology. Vomiting is controlled by the vomiting centre (VC) located in the medulla. It may be activated by stimuli from the chemoreceptor trigger zone (sensitive to chemical stimuli), the upper gastrointestinal tract and pharynx, the vestibular apparatus and higher cortical centres (Figure 3.1). The vomiting centre co-ordinates the act of vomiting via autonomic efferents to the gastrointestinal tract. Interaction with other brain stem centres produces the associated autonomic features (pallor, sweating, salivation and tachycardia). Co-ordination with the respiratory centre facilitates breath holding and the forceful contraction of the respiratory muscles which causes vomiting.

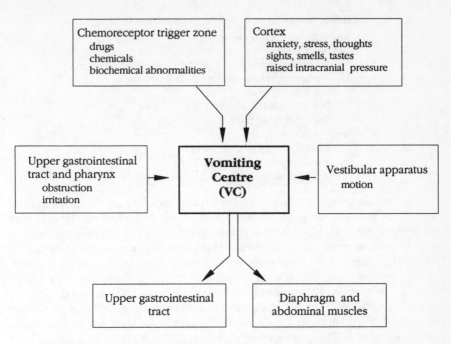

Figure 3.1 Diagrammatic representation of the mechanism of vomiting

Cause (Table 3.10). Patients with cancer frequently have multiple causes for nausea and vomiting.

Table 3.10 Causes of nausea and vomiting

via peripheral afferent	*via chemoreceptor trigger zone*
irritation, obstruction of the gastrointestinal tract	biochemical abnormalities
(including pharynx and hepatobiliary system)	hypercalcemia
cancer	hyponatremia
chronic cough	liver failure, renal failure
esophagitis	sepsis
gastritis	drugs
peptic ulceration	chemotherapy
gastric distension	opioids, digoxin
gastric compression	antibiotics, other
delayed gastric emptying	*via vestibular system*
bowel obstruction	malignant vestibular infiltration
constipation	drugs : aspirin, platinum
hepatitis	*via cortical centres*
biliary obstruction	psychological factors, anxiety
chemotherapy	sights, smells, tastes
radiotherapy	conditioned vomiting
	raised intracranial pressure

Treatment

The principles of treatment are outlined in Table 3.11. The underlying cause is sought and treated whenever possible and clinically appropriate.

Table 3.11 Nausea and vomiting : principles of treatment
assess for and treat underlying cause
use of antiemetics
drug selected on basis of presumed causative mechanism
commence before vomiting starts if possible
in adequate doses
in combination if necessary
by parenteral or rectal route if necessary
if unresponsive
assess for psychological factors
reassess for missed physical causes
try different antiemetics and/or combinations

Antiemetic drugs. The antiemetic drugs in clinical use are described in Table 3.12. Where possible, antiemetics are selected for use on the basis of the presumed causative mechanism for the nausea and vomiting. Nausea and vomiting mediated via the CTZ responds well to antiemetics with antidopaminergic action. Gastric stasis and compression respond to the gastrokinetic effect of metoclopramide or cisapride. A 5-HT$_3$ receptor antagonist is used for patients receiving chemotherapy or radiotherapy. Cortical causes of nausea and vomiting may respond to anxiolytic drugs. If the condition does not respond satisfactorily to treatment, a trial of different antiemetic drugs or combinations may be successful. Common side effects include extrapyramidal (Table 3.13) and anticholinergic effects (Table 3.14).

Table 3.13 Extrapyramidal side effects

acute dystonic reactions	
onset	within days of starting oral therapy, within minutes of IV injection
features	trismus, torticollis, facial spasm, oculogyric crisis, opisthotonus, anxiety
treatment	benztropine 1-2 mg IV or IM *or* diphenhydramine 25-50 mg IV or IM
akathisia	
onset	within weeks of starting oral therapy, within minutes of IV injection
features	motor restlessness, compulsive moving, anxiety
treatment	as for acute dystonic reactions
Parkinsonism	
onset	usually after several weeks of therapy
features	intention tremor, muscular rigidity, bradykinesia
treatment	discontinue causative agent; benztropine or procyclidine
tardive dyskinesia	
onset	usually after months of treatment
features	involuntary chewing movements, vermicular movements of tongue
treatment	discontinue causative agent

Table 3.14 Anticholinergic side effects

dry mouth (xerostomia)
blurred vision (mydriasis and loss of accommodation)
difficulty with micturition, retention
constipation
reflux esophagitis
tachycardia, palpitations
anhidrosis, fever
acute confusion or delirium

Table 3.12 The antiemetic agents

phenothiazines	prochlorperazine, chlorpromazine
action	antidopaminergic effect at the CTZ
side effects	EP (prochlorperazine), sedation and hypotension (chlorpromazine)
butyrophenone	haloperidol
action	antidopaminergic effect at the CTZ
side effects	sedation and EP
orthopromides	metoclopramide
action	antidopaminergic effect at the CTZ and direct gastrokinetic effect
precaution	may aggravate high small bowel obstruction
side effects	sedation and EP
anticholinergic	scopolamine hydrobromide
action	anticholinergic effect at or near the VC, reduces GI secretions and motility
side effects	whole spectrum of anticholinergic effects
antihistamine	diphenhydramine, cyclizine
action	at VC by an uncertain mechanism
use	will potentiate antiemetic effect of a dopamine antagonist and prevent EP
side effects	side effects include sedation and dryness of the mouth
cannabinoid	dronabinol
action	at a cortical level : the antiemetic effect parallels the euphoric period
side effects	drowsiness, dysphoria and delusions (worse in older patients)
corticosteroids	prednisolone, dexamethasone, hydrocortisone
action	undefined mechanism
use	particular value for vomiting associated with raised intracranial pressure
benzodiazepines	diazepam, lorazepam
action	at a cortical level
use	used with other antiemetics for patients receiving chemotherapy
5HT$_3$ antagonists	ondansetron, granisetron
action	prevent vagal stimulation in GI tract; may also have central action
use	vomiting associated with chemotherapy, radiotherapy
side effects	constipation, headache
prokinetic agent	cisapride
action	acetylcholine release in the myenteric plexus increases GI peristalsis
side effects	colic, diarrhoea

CTZ – chemoreceptor trigger zone, EP–extrapyramidal side effects, GI– gastrointestinal, VC–vomiting centre

Terminal care. During the last days or week of life, treatment directed at an underlying cause may be inappropriate. Symptomatic treatment with antiemetics is continued and the use of drugs with sedative side effects may be valuable. Some antiemetic drugs can be given by the rectal route and metoclopramide and haloperidol can be included in syringe drivers used for subcutaneous infusions of morphine. Nasogastric intubation should be avoided.

HICCUPS

Hiccups are due to involuntary contraction of the diaphragm causing sudden inspiration associated with glottic closure.

Cause. Hiccups are most frequently caused by diaphragmatic irritation or gastric distension (Table 3.15). A patient with protracted or distressing hiccups should have a chest x-ray and a serum creatinine estimation performed.

Treatment

If hiccups occur only intermittently or for short periods, no treatment may be necessary except perhaps for one of the 'home cures' (Table 3.16). Protracted

Table 3.15 Causes of hiccups

diaphragmatic irritation
    malignant infiltration
    inflammation or infection : empyema, pleurodesis, subphrenic abscess
    marked hepatomegaly, ascites
gastric distension or obstruction
    obstruction, overload, gastric tumor
esophagitis
phrenic nerve irritation
    mediastinal tumor
intracranial disease
    cerebral or medullary tumor
metabolic
    uremia

unresponsive hiccups are treated with chlorpromazine. This will cause some sedation and postural hypotension but is usually effective in stopping an attack. Other drugs reported to be of benefit include baclofen and nifedipine.

Terminal care. Relief of gastric distension may improve the patient's comfort as well as stopping hiccups. Otherwise, troublesome hiccups during the terminal phase should be treated with chlorpromazine.

Table 3.16 Management of hiccups

to abort an attack	
vagal, pharyngeal stimulation	pharyngeal stimulation : swab, nasogastric tube
	massage external auditory meatus
	sneezing
	drinking from 'wrong' side of the glass
elevation of pCO_2	breath holding, rebreathing into paper bag
reduction of gastric distension	aerated drink, peppermint water
	metoclopramide, cisapride
	nasogastric tube
pharmacological	chlorpromazine 25-50 mg IV, PO
to prevent further attacks	
treat underlying cause	
hiccups due to intracranial disease	phenytoin, carbamazepine
treatment of gastric distension	as above; surgery
pharmacological	chlorpromazine 10-25 mg PO q6h

DYSPHAGIA

Dysphagia is difficulty with swallowing.

Cause (Table 3.17).

Clinical features. With abnormalities of the buccal phase, food stays in the mouth and there is often drooling. With pharyngeal dysphagia, food sticks in the throat and attempts at swallowing cause gagging, coughing and regurgitation of food through the nose. Patients with esophageal disorders complain that food sticks somewhere behind the sternum.

Obstruction caused by tumor usually causes dysphagia which is initially more marked for solids than liquids; dysphagia due to neuromuscular pathology affects solids and fluids to much the same extent.

Table 3.17 Causes of dysphagia

buccal phase – *food voluntarily pushed backward by the tongue and palate*
    tumor : intrinsic obstruction, functional deficit
    stomatitis : infections, radiation, chemotherapy
    xerostomia
    neuromuscular dysfunction : surgery, cranial nerve dysfunction, cerebral or brain stem
        lesions, general weakness and debility
pharyngeal phase – *swallowing reflex initiated, including glottic closure*
    tumor : intrinsic obstruction, extrinsic compression
    pharyngitis : infection, radiation
    neuromuscular dysfunction : surgery, cranial nerve dysfunction, cerebral or brain stem
        lesions, general weakness or debility, radiation fibrosis or stricture
esophageal phase – *food passed down the esophagus by reflex peristalsis*
    tumor : intrinsic obstruction, extrinsic compression
    esophagitis : infection, radiation, reflux
    neuromuscular dysfunction : surgery, mural plexus infiltration, radiation fibrosis or stricture,
        anxiety

Assessment. Examination includes testing cranial nerve function and inspection of the oropharynx for evidence of tumor or infection. Swallowing may be assessed radiologically using a dilute barium solution. Patients with esophageal dysphagia require a chest x-ray or CT scan to assess mediastinal disease and endoscopy is used to differentiate intrinsic pathology and extrinsic pressure.

Treatment

Oropharyngeal dysphagia. The treatment options are set out in Table 3.18. Patients with oropharyngeal dysphagia require a program of feeding education, including assistance with positioning to make swallowing easier and dietary advice about small meals and soft moist food. The accumulation of saliva in patients with complete obstruction will cause drooling and may lead to aspiration; treatment is with an anticholinergic drug to reduce salivary flow.

Table 3.18 Dysphagia : some treatment options

buccal and pharyngeal	
obstructing tumor	surgery, laser resection, radiotherapy
extrinsic compression	corticosteroids, radiotherapy
neuromuscular inco-ordination	corticosteroids, radiotherapy
stomatitis, pharyngitis, xerostomia	standard therapy (see Tables 3.2, 3.5)
general	feeding education, dietary advice, enteral nutrition
esophageal	
esophagitis	standard therapy (see Table 3.20)
chronic stricture	dilatation
neuromuscular inco-ordination	dietary advice, corticosteroids
extrinsic compression	corticosteroids, radiotherapy, systemic therapy
intrinsic tumor	endo-esophageal tube
	radiotherapy, systemic therapy
	endoscopic laser resection

Enteral nutrition. Patients with severe oropharyngeal dysphagia may require feeding by an alternative route. Long-term nasogastric intubation should be avoided and the endoscopic placement of a percutaneous gastrostomy tube under local anesthetic is the preferred approach. It has a low complication rate but is not suitable for patients with ascites, peptic ulceration or a bleeding diathesis.

Esophageal obstruction. Esophageal obstruction due to tumor may respond temporarily to corticosteroids and radiotherapy may be considered. Endoscopic laser resection is the treatment of choice for intrinsic tumor when technically feasible. It has the advantage that the relief of dysphagia is immediate (compared to one to a few weeks following radiotherapy) and the procedure can be repeated as often as clinically required.

Endo-esophageal tubes. An endo-esophageal tube (e.g. Celestin, Atkinson) can be placed either endoscopically or via a small upper abdominal incision; the latter procedure is preferred as a larger tube can be inserted and sewn into position to prevent dislodgment. Intubation provides immediate relief of dysphagia but may also allow relatively free gastroesophageal reflux. The patient's diet is initially liquid, progressing slowly to a semisolid or solid diet by the end of a week. Patients are advised to take multiple small meals accompanied by an aerated drink. Foods which are likely to cause obstruction of the tube, such as lumpy or stringy foods and fresh bread, are avoided. If blockage occurs, the patient can try to clear the tube with an aerated drink or with physical movement. Endoscopic clearance is sometimes necessary.

Terminal care. Patients with oropharyngeal dysphagia should be managed conservatively with dietary manipulation. An endo-esophageal tube should be considered for complete esophageal obstruction as insertion causes little distress and it may greatly improve the quality of life if it allows saliva to be swallowed.

ESOPHAGITIS

Cause (Table 3.19).

Table 3.19 Causes of esophagitis

tumor infiltration	
radiation	predisposition to infection, peptic irritation
chemotherapy	neutropenia
infection	fungal, bacterial, viral
reflux esophagitis	raised intra-abdominal pressure (any cause)
	endo-esophageal tubes
	nasogastric tube
	prolonged recumbent posture
	persistent vomiting
	anticholinergic drugs, anticholinergic side effects of drugs

Clinical features. Esophagitis causes pain on swallowing (odynophagia), some degree of difficulty with swallowing (dysphagia) and may produce angina-like mediastinal pain. Severe esophagitis may result in blood stained vomitus or melena.

Assessment. Examination may show oropharyngeal infection or evidence of raised intra-abdominal pressure. Barium examination will show mucosal irregularity or ulceration. Endoscopy with biopsies and cultures may be required.

Treatment

Therapy is directed at pain relief, prevention and healing of ulceration, control of reflux, treatment of infection and, where possible, treatment of the underlying cause (Table 3.20). Topical local anesthetics in combination with antacids often provide good symptom relief. However, the topical local anesthetics such as lidocaine or cocaine may predispose to aspiration if the pharynx is anesthetized. The use of an H_2-receptor antagonist or acid pump inhibitor to reduce gastric acid production may significantly aid analgesia.

Terminal care. The treatment of esophagitis should be purely symptomatic. Elevating the head of the bed, topical anesthetics, combined antacids and dietary manipulation are helpful. Parenteral opioid analgesics are given for severe pain.

Table 3.20 Management of esophagitis

pain relief
 topical local anesthetics : lidocaine, cocaine
 oral analgesics (mild), parenteral opioids (severe)
 antacids
 dietary advice : liquid or semisolid diet, avoid very hot or cold foods
prevention and healing of ulceration
 antacids combined with coating agent alginate
 sucralfate
reduce gastric acid production : H_2-receptor antagonist, acid pump inhibitor
avoidance of reflux
 reduce increased intra-abdominal pressure
 dietary : avoid large meals, carbonated drinks, alcohol
 posture : avoid stooping, lying flat
 increase lower esophageal sphincter tone : metoclopramide, cisapride
infection
 specific antimicrobial therapy

UPPER GASTROINTESTINAL BLEEDING

Cause (Table 3.21).

Table 3.21 Causes of upper gastrointestinal bleeding

esophagus
 esophagitis, malignant infiltration, esophageal varices, Mallory Weiss tears
stomach and duodenum
 erosion, ulceration, malignant infiltration
general bleeding diathesis

Clinical features. Upper gastrointestinal hemorrhage may cause the vomiting of blood or 'coffee grounds' and is usually associated with melena. If the hemorrhage is mild and chronic, there may be no hematemesis or melena but simply a slowly developing anemia.

Assessment. Endoscopy will define the cause of bleeding in the majority of patients providing the procedure is appropriate to the stage of the disease. Endoscopy will allow visualization of tumor, demonstration of multiple sites of bleeding and identification of patients likely to continue to bleed or re-bleed. Endoscopy may also provide the opportunity for topical treatment.

Treatment

Management includes treatment of the cause, blood transfusion if indicated and the correction of any bleeding diathesis (Table 3.22). If endoscopy is not performed the patient may be treated symptomatically with transfusion and given empiric therapy for the presumed cause of bleeding. The temporary use of a Sengstaken tube may be considered for acute variceal bleeding but would be inappropriate for terminally ill patients.

Table 3.22 Upper gastrointestinal bleeding : treatment options

erosions and peptic ulceration
    withdraw causative or aggravating agent
    antacids, sucralfate, H$_2$-receptor antagonist, acid pump inhibitor, misoprostol
    local photocoagulation, electrocoagulation (if vessels visualized)
bleeding varices
    endoscopic sclerotherapy
    vasopressin 0.5 ml or 10 units IM or SC
    octreotide infusion (25 µg/h IV)
bleeding tumors
    laser photocoagulation
    electrocoagulation, sclerotherapy (if vessels visualized)
    surgery, embolization

> *Treatment must be appropriate to the stage of the patient's disease and the prognosis*

Terminal care. Treatment is symptomatic with antiemetics and analgesics. Antacids and therapy to reduce gastric acid production can be continued if they aid pain control and administration does not distress the patient. Parenteral morphine, given to allay anxiety, may be considered for patients who suffer massive or repeated hematemeses.

INDIGESTION

Indigestion is variously used to describe epigastric fullness, discomfort and pain, sometimes associated with bloating or distension, flatulence and belching, nausea or symptoms of esophageal reflux.
    Cause (Table 3.23).

Table 3.23 Causes of indigestion

esophagus : esophagitis
stomach and duodenum
    cancer
    gastritis : radiotherapy, chemotherapy, alcohol, drugs
    erosions and peptic ulceration : aspirin, NSAIDs, alcohol
    small stomach syndrome : gastrectomy, linitis plastica
    gastric compression syndrome : hepatomegaly, splenomegaly, ascites
    gastric outlet obstruction : tumor, peptic ulceration, opioid drugs
    dumping syndrome : gastrectomy
    aerophagia : anxiety, pharyngeal abnormalities
pancreas : pancreatitis, pancreatic cancer
biliary system : cholecystitis, cancer

Clinical features. The syndromes relating to an effective reduction in stomach size or its inability to expand with feeding are characterized by early satiety and inability to eat large amounts. There is epigastric discomfort often associated with nausea and symptoms of esophageal reflux. The dumping syndrome, caused by the rapid transit of food out of the stomach in patients who have had a partial gastrectomy or vagotomy, is characterized by epigastric discomfort and fullness associated with nausea, colic and diarrhea accompanied by vasomotor symptoms of weakness, faintness and sweating.
    Assessment. The characteristics of the pain and other associated clinical features often indicate the probable cause but endoscopy is frequently required to diagnose mucosal lesions.

Treatment

The management of dyspepsia includes measures to relieve symptoms, withdrawal of offending drugs and treatment of underlying or predisposing factors. A variety of medications may be employed (Table 3.24).

Table 3.24 Indigestion : medications

antacids
action symptomatic relief by neutralization of gastric acid
side effects aluminum hydroxide : constipation, drug malabsorption
  magnesium salts : diarrhea, hypermagnesemia (in renal failure)
  sodium bicarbonate : sodium overload, metabolic alkalosis
  calcium carbonate : constipation, rebound hyperacidity
combined antacids
action with simethicone : facilitates expulsion of wind
  with alginic acid : provides a protective mucosal coating
mucosal protective agent : sucralfate
action forms a protective mucosal coating; aids ulcer healing
given at least 30 minutes after antacids and 2 hours after H_2-receptor antagonists
H_2-receptor antagonists : cimetidine, ranitidine, famotidine, nizatidine
action reduce gastric acid production
side effects increased hepatic enzymes, drug interactions
acid pump inhibitors : omeprazole, lansoprazole
action prevents gastric acid secretion
side effects mild nausea and diarrhea
prostaglandin analogue : misoprostol
action synthetic prostaglandin analogue which inhibits gastric acid secretion
side effect diarrhea
gastrokinetic agents : metoclopramide, cisapride
action promote gastric emptying
side effects sedation, extrapyramidal effects (metoclopramide); colic, diarrhea (cisapride)

Gastric restriction syndromes. The treatment of the syndromes related to gastric restriction is symptomatic (Table 3.25). Gastrokinetic drugs are particularly useful for patients with obstruction caused by opioid analgesic or anticholinergic drugs which need to be continued.

Table 3.25 Indigestion : management

gastric restriction
  dietary advice : multiple small meals
  antiflatuent : simethicone-containing antacid
  gastrokinetic agent
  stop drugs causing gastric stasis/outlet obstruction, if possible
erosions and peptic ulceration
  sucralfate, H_2-receptor antagonist, acid pump inhibitor, misoprostol

Peptic ulceration. Peptic ulceration is initially treated with an H_2-receptor antagonist; omeprazole or other acid pump inhibitor is used if there is no response or if the condition developed despite prophylactic H_2-receptor antagonist therapy. An acid pump inhibitor or misoprostol will produce better results in patients taking NSAIDs, especially if the NSAID needs to be continued. Whenever possible, the treatment of acid peptic disease should be with medical measures although surgery may be required if there is obstruction, perforation or continued bleeding.

Preventive therapy. Patients given aspirin or NSAIDs should be considered for prophylactic therapy: antacids are ineffective but an H_2-receptor antagonist or sucralfate may reduce the incidence of duodenal and esophageal ulceration; an acid pump inhibitor and misoprostol may prevent gastric ulceration. If *Helicobacter pylori* infection is present, patients with longer life expectancy can be considered for eradication therapy.

Terminal care. Antacids can be continued to control symptoms. H_2-receptor antagonists or opioids can be used for pain not relieved by antacids.

BOWEL OBSTRUCTION

Cause (Table 3.26). Bowel obstruction in patients with advanced cancer is frequently due to more than one cause and obstruction often occurs at multiple sites in patients with peritoneal infiltration.

Table 3.26 Causes of bowel obstruction

mechanical obstruction
luminal obstruction : cancer, constipation, fecal impaction
wall infiltration, stricture formation : cancer, radiation, surgery, benign (peptic ulcer)
extrinsic compression : cancer, adhesions (surgical, malignant)
paralytic obstruction
disruption of autonomic nerve supply : retroperitoneal infiltration, spinal disease
drugs : opioids, anticholinergics
postoperative
peritonitis
metabolic : hypokalemia, hypercalcemia
radiation fibrosis
arterial or venous insufficiency

Clinical features. The classical features of bowel obstruction are abdominal pain and distension, nausea and vomiting, and failure to pass flatus or feces. The clinical features depend on whether the obstruction is acute or subacute, complete or partial, and which part of the bowel is involved. In patients with advanced cancer the obstruction is more likely to be incomplete and subacute. The higher the obstruction, the earlier and more profuse the vomiting; lower obstruction is associated with more abdominal distension. Patients with fecal impaction may pass fecal material which is an overflow phenomenon. Plain x-rays will show distended bowel with fluid levels on the erect or decubitus view.

Treatment

The management of bowel obstruction is traditionally based on surgical intervention but conservative therapy may produce equivalent results in some patients with advanced cancer. The options available are listed in Table 3.27.

Nasogastric intubation and intravenous fluids. Nasogastric drainage with intravenous fluid administration should be used as a temporary measure only. Patients with advanced cancer are more likely to have incomplete and subacute obstructions, many of which will resolve spontaneously. They should be managed with symptomatic treatment as described below and not with chronic nasogastric intubation.

Surgery. The clinical features which recommend surgical intervention are listed in Table 3.28. A significant proportion of patients (estimated at between 10 and 30%) will have a benign and correctable cause. The majority of patients who undergo

Table 3.27 Bowel obstruction : treatment options

nasogastric intubation and intravenous fluids as a temporary measure only
    preoperative
    pending a decision regarding surgery
    while systemic therapy is initiated
    acute phase of recurrent obstruction

> *Treatment must be appropriate to the stage of the patient's disease and the prognosis*

surgery
    resection or bypass of obstruction
    creation of colostomy, ileostomy
    percutaneous gastrostomy
    endoscopic laser resection (colorectal)

symptomatic
    medications (see Table 3.29)
    relieve and prevent constipation
    general : small meals with reduced roughage
                   served early in the day or when the patient requests

surgery for bowel obstruction do not re-obstruct even though the cancer continues to progress. However, there is an operative mortality and a few patients will have postoperative fecal fistulas. Except for the terminally ill, urgent surgery must be considered for patients with peritonitis.

Patients with gastric outlet obstruction are less likely to respond to symptomatic management. Creation of a gastroenterostomy or the use of a percutaneous gastrostomy as a venting procedure should be considered for patients with a high complete obstruction whose nausea and vomiting are otherwise difficult to control.

Colorectal obstruction due to luminal tumor may be treated with endoscopic laser resection. The procedure is well tolerated and preferable to a colostomy.

Table 3.28 Bowel obstruction : management guidelines

	bowel obstruction	
acute ± complete		subacute ± intermittent ± incomplete
peritonitis		no focal signs
		multiple palpable masses
strangulated hernia		
gastric outlet obstruction		
first episode of obstruction		multiple episodes of obstruction
previous benign obstruction		
previous radiotherapy		
previous surgical findings do not preclude successful surgery		previous surgical findings preclude successful surgery
younger fitter patient		older ± more debilitated
other systemic therapy available		no systemic therapy available
patient's consent		patient declines surgery
↓		↓
favor earlier surgical intervention		favor symptomatic management

Table 3.29   Symptomatic treatment of bowel obstruction : examples of medications used

antiemetics			
prochlorperazine	5-10 mg PO q6h	*or*	25 mg PR q6h
metoclopramide	10 mg PO q4-6h	*or*	40-60 mg/24h SC infusion
haloperidol	0.5-1 mg PO q6h	*or*	3-5 mg/24h SC infusion
analgesics			
morphine PO, PR or SC infusion			
anticholinergics			
scopolamine hydrobromide	0.4 mg SC q6h	*or*	0.6-1.2 mg/24h SC infusion
somatostatin analogue			
octreotide	0.1 mg SC q8h	*or*	0.2-0.3 mg/24h SC infusion
corticosteroid			
dexamethasone	8-16 mg/d PO	*or*	8-16 mg/24h SC infusion

Symptomatic management. Symptomatic management of nausea, vomiting and pain will benefit many patients for whom surgery is considered inappropriate (Table 3.29). Nausea and vomiting are reduced to a minimum; for some patients with chronic obstruction, vomiting once or twice a day may be 'well tolerated' and preferred to a nasogastric tube.   The gastrokinetic antiemetic drug metoclopramide is contraindicated for patients with high small bowel obstruction as it may aggravate vomiting. Cisapride has a prokinetic effect on the whole bowel and may be used if there is no physical obstruction. Anticholinergic drugs reduce gastrointestinal secretions and lessen nausea, vomiting and colic.   Octreotide reduces gastrointestinal secretions and motility and can control refractory vomiting in patients with bowel obstruction. Corticosteroids benefit some patients with chronic bowel obstruction.   Additional measures include the treatment and prevention of constipation and a dietary program of small meals with reduced roughage.

Terminal care. Treatment is symptomatic with analgesic, antiemetic and anticholinergic drugs. Surgical considerations are usually inappropriate. Nasogastric tubes and intravenous lines are undignified and unnecessary.

CONSTIPATION

Constipation refers to infrequent or difficult defecation. It is the passage of a reduced number of bowel actions, which may or may not be abnormally hard, with increased difficulty. Constipation implies a significant variation from the normal bowel habit for an individual patient.

Cause (Table 3.30). The etiology of constipation is frequently multifactorial and many drugs used in palliative care predispose to constipation.

Clinical features. Constipation varies from a reduction in the number or frequency of bowel actions in an otherwise asymptomatic patient to complete cessation with the symptoms and signs of fecal impaction. Stools may be abnormally hard, although constipation may occur with normal or soft stools in those with neurological disability. Patients with fecal impaction can present complaining of diarrhea and continue to pass fecal material as an overflow phenomenon. Anorexia, nausea and vomiting frequently accompany severe constipation.

Assessment. The clinical assessment of constipation is summarized in Table 3.31 Further investigations are rarely necessary except for a plain x-ray to exclude bowel obstruction.

Table 3.30 Causes of constipation

general	*colorectal*
immobility, inactivity	obstruction
muscular weakness, debility	pelvic tumor mass
confusion, sedation	radiation fibrosis, stricture
fear of bedpans	painful anorectal conditions
inability to access or use	*drugs*
toilet facility	opioid analgesics
nutritional	antidiarrheals
decreased intake	non-opioid analgesics
low residue diet	anticholinergic drugs or side effects
poor fluid intake	anticholinergics
metabolic	antispasmodics
dehydration	antidepressants
hypercalcemia	phenothiazines
hypokalemia	haloperidol
uremia	antacids
neurological	antiemetics
cerebral tumor	ondansetron
spinal cord disease	anticancer
sacral nerve root infiltration	vinca alkaloids
psychological	diuretics
depression	other
fear of diarrhea, incontinence	iron, barium

Table 3.31 Assessment of constipation

information required

pattern of patient's recent bowel movements
pattern of patient's pre-illness bowel movements
  previous long term use of laxatives

use of potentially constipating drugs
use of laxatives and their effect

patient's food intake and its fiber content
patient's fluid intake

presence or absence of feces in the rectum
consistency of feces - soft or hard

presence of anal tone, reflex
sacral nerve root sensation

underlying cause - usually multiple
stage of patient's disease and prognosis

Treatment

General measures. An adequate fluid intake is important in the prevention and treatment of constipation. Patients are encouraged to take food or fluids which have some laxative properties, such as fruit and prune juice. In the absence of intestinal obstruction, foods with a high fiber content are encouraged, but the amount of fiber should be increased slowly as large amounts are often poorly tolerated by elderly or debilitated patients.

Lack of easy access to toilet facilities, or the ready availability of assistance to use them, can cause or aggravate constipation especially for the elderly or frail. An elevated toilet seat makes it easier for the patient to get on and off the toilet, and a foot stool facilitates the use of leg and abdominal muscles in the act of defecation.

Laxatives. Laxatives are the mainstay of the treatment of constipation in palliative care. A number of different laxatives are commercially available and it is necessary to know what a patient has been taking, successfully or unsuccessfully. The different mechanisms of action of the various laxatives are listed in Table 3.32.

Table 3.32 Laxatives and suppositories

bulk forming laxatives

includes	psyllium (Metamucil), methylcellulose, dietary fiber supplements
action	retention of intraluminal fluid → softens feces and stimulates peristalsis
precautions	patients must drink extra fluids; unsuitable for elderly, debilitated
side effects	unpalatable, colic, flatulence (considerable individual variation)

lubricant laxatives

includes	mineral oil
action	lubricant and fecal softener
side effects	lipoid pneumonia if aspirated

fecal softener

includes	docusate
action	fecal softener; also promotes secretion of fluid into bowel

contact (stimulant) laxatives

includes	polyphenolics : phenolphthalein, bisacodyl
	anthracenes : senna, cascara
action	promote secretion of fluid → softens feces and stimulates peristalsis
side effects	dehydration and electrolyte imbalance in debilitated patients

osmotic laxatives

includes	magnesium salts : sulfate (Epsom salts), hydroxide (milk of magnesia)
	nonabsorbable sugars : lactulose, sorbitol, mannitol, polyethylene glycol
action	draws fluid into bowel by osmosis → softens feces and stimulates peristalsis
precautions	patient must drink extra fluids; unsuitable for elderly, debilitated
side effects	colic, flatulence (considerable individual variation),
	dehydration and electrolyte imbalance in debilitated patients

rectal suppositories

includes	glycerin, bisacodyl
action	fecal softener (glycerin), contact or stimulant (bisacodyl)
use	glycerin inserted into fecal matter, bisacodyl against mucosa

Suppositories. Rectally administered laxatives (Table 3.32) are used to initiate evacuation of the lower bowel while awaiting the effect of orally administered medications. Regular use should be unnecessary except in patients with a neurogenic bowel.

Enemas. Enemas are used to relieve constipation if suppositories are ineffective. Small volume enemas are less distressing for the patient and easier to use in the home environment. For more difficult constipation, sodium phosphate enemas can be used but may cause fluid and electrolyte imbalance in debilitated or dehydrated patients. Soap and water enemas may cause fluid overload and should be discouraged. For refractory constipation an olive oil retention enema given overnight may be successful.

Prevention of constipation. The factors which predispose to constipation are well known and prophylactic treatment should be introduced before clinical problems develop (Table 3.33). This is particularly important for patients taking morphine or other opioid drugs.

Table 3.33 Prophylaxis of constipation

initial assessment	laxatives
recent bowel action pattern	docusate 240-480 mg nocte
pre-illness bowel action pattern	*or* bisacodyl 10-20 mg nocte
recent use and effect of laxatives	± senna 15 mg nocte
use of other constipating drugs	± lactulose 30 ml nocte
general measures (where feasible)	and titrate the dose against the clinical effect
increased food intake	explanation to patient, family
increased dietary fiber	treatment of painful rectal conditions
or bulk forming laxative	ensure access and ability to use toilet facilities
increased fluid intake	avoid constipating drugs if possible
encourage activity	keep a record of bowel actions

Treatment of established constipation. The treatment of established constipation requires the use of suppositories and enemas to clear the lower bowel before a normal bowel pattern can be established with oral medication (Table 3.34). Patients with fecal impaction may require manual disimpaction which is performed with appropriate analgesia and sedation.

Table 3.34 Management of constipation

initial assessment (Table 3.31)
rectal examination
  absent rectal tone, reflex or sensation : neurogenic bowel (see Table 3.35)
  no neurological abnormality
    feces in rectum
      hard feces : glycerin PR, microenema, enema (oil), disimpaction
      soft feces : bisacodyl PR, microenema, enema, disimpaction
    empty rectum → plain x-ray
      no bowel obstruction : bisacodyl PR, oral medications
      bowel obstruction   : appropriate treatment
institute a program of prevention (Table 3.33)

Management of neurogenic bowel. The aim of bowel care is to evacuate the bowel every one or two days (depending on previous bowel habit) and at night or morning depending on what is most convenient for the patient (Table 3.35).

Table 3.35 Management of neurogenic bowel

spinal cord lesion – *spastic bowel, hypertonic anal sphincter, sacral reflexes intact*
  adequate fluid and fiber intake
  oral laxatives (avoid laxatives which cause excessive softening)
  rectal suppositories or stimulation leads to increased peristalsis and sphincter relaxation
sacral nerve root lesion – *reduced peristalsis, flaccid sphincter, sacral reflexes absent*
  adequate fluid and fiber intake
  oral laxatives
  rectal suppositories or stimulation may lead to evacuation
  straining and abdominal massage
  cholinergic drugs (e.g. bethanechol 10 mg PO q8h)

Terminal care. Significant symptoms due to constipation are rare during the last days or week of life. Oral intake of food and fluid is frequently limited and laxatives can usually be discontinued. A suppository or microenema can be used if the patient has pain, feels the urge to defecate but is unable to do so, or if there is continued fecal incontinence due to impaction.

DIARRHEA

Diarrhea is an increase in the frequency and fluidity of bowel actions. Diarrhea implies a significant variation from the normal pattern of bowel movements for a particular patient.

Cause (Table 3.36). More than one mechanism is frequently involved. Diarrhea occurs when there is increased fecal water, caused by either increased secretion or reduced absorption. The amount of water is greater than can be absorbed by the bowel distal to the site of production or the resorptive process is short-circuited by a surgical or malignant fistula. Osmotic diarrhea occurs when increased amounts of water are drawn into the bowel by increased solute loads or laxatives. Secretory diarrhea, with enhanced formation of gastrointestinal secretions, occurs with infection, inflammation and the hormone-related syndromes.

Table 3.36 Causes of diarrhea

dietary	inflammation
excess roughage, fiber	radiation, drugs
nasogastric feeding	steatorrhea (fat malabsorption)
enteric supplements	pancreatic insufficiency
drugs	biliary obstruction, exclusion
laxatives	bacterial overgrowth
magnesium antacids	bile salt malabsorption
misoprostol	ileal resection or bypass
antibiotics, cytotoxics, others	bacterial overgrowth
surgical	hormonal
gastrectomy, vagotomy	carcinoid
enterocolic anastomosis	Zollinger-Ellison syndrome
cancer	medullary carcinoma of thyroid
gastrocolic fistula	VIPoma and others
enterocolic fistula	psychological
hemorrhage	anxiety
infection	obstruction with overflow
pseudomembranous colitis	fecal impaction
blind loops	rectal tumor

Assessment. The cause is usually evident from the history and clinical examination which includes rectal examination and inspection of the stool. Other investigations may be considered if the results will significantly affect treatment decisions.

Treatment

General measures. Maintenance of hydration is important except in the terminally ill. Commercially available soft drinks or oral rehydration solutions can be used. Intravenous rehydration may be necessary if diarrhea is severe or if there is vomiting. Dietary modifications to both reduce diarrhea and ensure adequate nutrition are important; the assistance of a dietician is useful.

Treatment of the underlying cause. The underlying cause is treated, where possible (Table 3.37).

Table 3.37   Treatment of selected underlying causes of diarrhea

dietary : dietary modification, more dilute enteric feeding
drugs : adjust, withdraw
gastrectomy, vagotomy : small frequent meals
infection
    pseudomembranous colitis : vancomycin 125 mg q6h *or* metronidazole 400 mg q8h
    bacterial overgrowth : tetracycline 250 mg q6h *or* metronidazole 400 mg q8h
inflammation
    radiation : low residue diet, aspirin or NSAID, sucralfate
steatorrhea
    obstructive jaundice : appropriate therapy (see Table 3.52)
    ileal resection, bypass : cholestyramine 12-16 g/d, low fat diet
    pancreatic insufficiency : enzyme supplements, H_2 receptor antagonist, dietary advice
hormonal
    Zollinger-Ellison : omeprazole
    carcinoid : cyproheptadine, octreotide
    VIPoma : octreotide

> *Treatment must be appropriate to the stage of the patient's disease and the prognosis.*

Antidiarrheal agents. Medications used in the treatment of diarrhea are listed in Table 3.38. Unless morphine or codeine are being given for analgesia, loperamide is the agent of choice. It is more effective than diphenoxylate or codeine, has few side effects and does not cause central nervous system depression.

Terminal care. Diarrhea should be controlled with oral loperamide or, for patients not taking oral medication, subcutaneous morphine. Investigations and energetic rehydration are inappropriate.

Table 3.38   Antidiarrheal agents

absorbent agents
   include   hydrophilic bulking agents e.g. methylcellulose, psyllium
   action   absorption of excess fluid
adsorbent agents
   include   kaolin preparations
   action   adsorption of bacteria, toxins and excess fluid
prostaglandin inhibitors
   include   aspirin, NSAIDs (excepting mefenamic acid, indomethacin)
   action   reduction in gastrointestinal secretions by inhibition of prostaglandin synthesis
   use   radiation enteritis
opioids
   include   loperamide, diphenoxylate, codeine
   action   inhibition of peristalsis
   use   loperamide : 4 mg initially, 2-4 mg q8-12h or after unformed motion, up to 16 mg/d
                diphenoxylate (2.5 mg with atropine 25 µg) : 5-10 mg initially, 2.5-5.0 mg q4-8h or after unformed motion, up to 20 mg/d
                codeine : 15-60 mg q4h
   side effects loperamide : few significant side effects, no CNS depression
                diphenoxylate : CNS depression may occur at doses >20 mg/d
                codeine : nausea, sedation and CNS depression at higher doses

FECAL INCONTINENCE, RECTAL DISCHARGE

Cause (Table 3.39). Fecal incontinence can occur with any cause of diarrhea, especially if the diarrhea is severe or the patient weak.

Table 3.39   Causes of faecal incontinence and rectal discharge

diarrhoea	rectovesical and rectovaginal fistulas
fecal impaction with overflow	neurogenic
rectal tumors	spinal cord lesions
proctitis	sacral nerve root lesions
rectal or pelvic surgery	

Assessment. Clinical assessment usually indicates the cause. Rectal examination will disclose impaction, rectal disease or neurological abnormalities. Further investigations are rarely necessary.

Treatment

Treatment is directed at the cause (Table 3.40). Special measures are taken to protect the perianal and perineal skin. After washing, the skin is patted dry with a soft cloth and dusted with zinc stearate or baby powder. If the skin is inflamed, hydrocortisone cream can be used for a few days, but may predispose to maceration and fungal infection. Ointments and creams are avoided as they will tend to keep the skin moist. Patients with fecal incontinence often feel ashamed and need reassurance that it is not their fault and that the ward staff understand it is due to their illness.

Table 3.40   Treatment of fecal incontinence, rectal discharge

diarrhea	appropriate therapy (see Diarrhea)
fecal impaction	appropriate therapy (see Constipation)
local tumor	diathermy, laser, radiotherapy, surgery
proctitis	corticosteroids (PR or PO), antibiotics

Neurogenic incontinence. For patients with a spinal cord lesion and a reasonable life expectancy, a program of bowel training is initiated (see Table 3.35). Patients with a shorter life expectancy or with sacral nerve root damage, for whom bowel retraining is not feasible, require a different approach. Dietary fiber is reduced and bulk laxatives avoided. Constipation is induced using codeine or loperamide, and regular bowel evacuations are planned once or twice a week using suppositories (if successful) or enemas.

Terminal care. If present, fecal impaction should be treated; in other situations it is probably best to induce a constipated state. Troublesome discharge due to proctitis is treated with corticosteroids.

PERIANAL AND VULVAL PRURITUS

Cause (Table 3.41). The cause is usually evident on clinical assessment.

Treatment. Treatment is that of the cause together with scrupulous skin hygiene, as described above for incontinent patients. Ointments and creams are best avoided as they will tend to keep the skin moist. Topical hydrocortisone cream can be used for a few days if irritation is severe. Zinc oxide paste will protect intact skin. Antipruritic lotions which may help are crotamiton (Eurax) and aluminum acetate (Burow's solution).

Table 3.41 Causes of pruritus ani and vulvae

infection
    candida, herpes simplex, condyloma acuminatum, bacterial
irradiation
malignant infiltration
poor local hygiene
incontinence, discharge
    rectal, vaginal, urinary
general
    generalized pruritus
    generalized dermatological condition

FLATULENCE

Gastric. Upper gastrointestinal flatulence is due to swallowed air. It is more common in people who are anxious, eat quickly or smoke. Behavioral modifications are usually successful. Other treatment include peppermint water, aerated drinks or simethicone, a defoaming agent which facilitates the bringing up of wind.

Intestinal. Intestinal gas is due to swallowed air and the chemical and bacterial degradation of food. Gas production will be increased by the ingestion of high fiber foods and nonabsorbable carbohydrates or with bacterial overgrowth of the small intestine. Increased intestinal gas production may cause distension, audible bowel sounds (borborygmi), painful colic and embarrassment at the noise and smell of wind passed. Dietary modifications or the use of an alternative laxative usually alleviate symptoms. Activated charcoal can reduce both the amount of flatus and the odor. Patients with small bowel bacterial overgrowth are treated with antibiotics.

LOWER GASTROINTESTINAL BLEEDING

Cause (Table 3.42).

Table 3.42 Causes of lower gastrointestinal bleeding

rectal	carcinoma
	proctitis : infection, radiotherapy, chemotherapy
	hemorrhoids
colonic	carcinoma
	colitis : infection, pseudomembranous colitis, radiotherapy
	diverticular disease
proximal	massive upper gastrointestinal bleeding
systemic	thrombocytopenia, coagulopathy

Treatment. The treatment is that of the cause. Unresectable tumors can be treated with diathermy, laser photocoagulation or radiotherapy. The topical application of 1% alum to bleeding rectal tumors may be of benefit. Proctitis and colitis are treated with topical or oral corticosteroids. Pseudomembranous colitis is treated with oral vancomycin.

STOMAS

Patients who are to have a colostomy or ileostomy created require preoperative counselling and postoperative training by a stomal therapist.

Skin care. Local inflammation and excoriation predispose to the appliance fitting poorly, which in turn leads to leakage and more skin damage. The peristomal skin is cleansed with water and mild soap; detergents, disinfectants and antiseptics cause irritation and dryness. A variety of preparations are available to protect skin, improve appliance adhesion and to allow healing of sore or broken skin. Severely inflamed peristomal skin can be treated with a corticosteroid cream or, if indicated by laboratory tests, a topical antibiotic. The area is then sealed with Opsite spray or similar sealant and the appliance fitted.

Other care. The management of diarrhea, constipation, flatus and odor are outlined in Table 3.43. Physical problems which may require treatment are listed in Table 3.44.

Table 3.43 Treatment of some ostomy related problems

diarrhea		*flatus and odor*
ileostomy	opioid antidiarrheal	dietary modification
colostomy	hydrophilic bulking agent	odor resistant disposable bags
	stop drugs causing diarrhea	deodorants added to bag
	dietary modification	charcoal filters
constipation		oral medications e.g. charcoal
colostomy	increase fluid intake	
	increase food, fiber	
	stop constipating drugs	
	laxative ± initial enema	

Table 3.44 Physical stomal problems : treatment options

obstruction	treat constipation, impaction, bowel obstruction
recession	treat conservatively unless there are continence problems; surgery
prolapse	manual reduction; surgery (not if intra-abdominal pressure raised)
parastomal herniation	treat conservatively unless there are continence problems; surgery
bleeding	topical sucralfate, 1% alum, silver nitrate; diathermy, laser
stomal recurrence	diathermy, laser; surgery if causing incontinence
perforation	use cone irrigation in preference to catheters

FISTULAS

Rectal. Rectovaginal and rectovesical fistulas are usually due to advanced pelvic disease and lead to passage of fecal material from the vagina or bladder. Creation of a defunctioning colostomy is the treatment of choice and provides complete relief. Terminally ill patients can be managed conservatively with reassurance, hygiene and skin care.

Enterocutaneous. Enterocutaneous fistulas usually develop as a complication of surgery. A small bowel fistula may produce copious amounts of fluid and the presence of digestive enzymes will cause skin damage. Management includes collection of the discharge in a bag or appliance, protection of the skin as set out in the section on stoma care, fluid and electrolyte replacement and measures to reduce the volume of drainage (Table 3 .45). A colonic fistula is managed in the same manner as a surgically created colostomy.

Table 3.45 Fistulas : drug treatment to reduce volume

loperamide	up to 4 mg PO q6h
scopolamine hydrobromide	0.4 mg SC q6h *or* 0.6-1.2 mg/24h SC infusion
octreotide	0.1 mg SC q8h *or* 0.2-0.3 mg/24h SC infusion

Buccal. Buccal fistulas between the mouth or pharynx and the face or neck will lead to leakage of saliva and ingested fluids. Small fistulas can be managed with regularly changed dry dressings. Larger fistulas may be improved with the use of plastic or silicone plugs, shaped or cast to the form of the fistula.

ASCITES

Cause (Table 3.46).

Table 3.46 Causes of ascites

peritoneal disease	venous obstruction
infiltration, infection, inflammation	cardiac failure
lymphatic obstruction	pericardial effusion, constriction
abdominal lymphatics, thoracic duct	inferior vena caval obstruction, thrombosis
hypoalbuminemia	hepatic vein obstruction, thrombosis
poor diet, liver disease	parenchymal liver disease
protein loss (repeated paracenteses)	portal vein obstruction, thrombosis

Assessment. In patients with cancer, the volume of fluid present is often considerable and investigations to confirm the presence of ascites are unnecessary. Smaller volumes can be detected on ultrasound or CT scanning.

Paracentesis is performed for diagnostic purposes. Ascites complicating primary liver disease and cardiac failure is clear and faintly amber. Carcinomatosis produces opaque straw colored fluid which may be blood stained. Chylous fluid, which indicates lymphatic obstruction, has a milky yellow or white appearance. The presence of malignant cells on cytological examination confirms peritoneal infiltration.

Treatment

Ascites due to malignant infiltration. Mild ascites which is neither progressive nor causing symptoms is managed with reassurance and observation. Systemic therapy should be considered for sensitive tumors as a response will lead to control of ascites. The other treatment options are listed in Table 3.47. Repeated paracentesis is appropriate for symptom control in the terminally ill and for ascites which reaccumulates very slowly, but is otherwise discouraged as it leads to protein depletion and predisposes to infection. Diuretic therapy benefits some patients but hydration and renal function need to be monitored. Instillation of sclerosants may inhibit reaccumulation but predisposes to loculation. A peritoneovenous shunt can be considered for patients with a reasonable life expectancy not responding to other therapy.

Chylous ascites. Chylous ascites is due to lymphatic obstruction in the high retroperitoneal region or the mediastinum. Repeated paracenteses will produce only transient improvement and intraperitoneal therapy is of no benefit. Radiotherapy can be employed if there is a demonstrable mass obstructing lymphatic flow in the mediastinum or retroperitoneum. Corticosteroids may also be of benefit.

Terminal care. Terminally ill patients who are symptomatic of ascites are managed by repeated paracentesis, performed as infrequently as possible.

Table 3.47 Management of ascites due to malignant infiltration

observation
systemic therapy (sensitive tumors)
paracentesis
    for diagnosis and initial symptom relief
    repeated paracentesis leads to protein depletion, infection
diuretics
    spironolactone 100 mg/d PO with furosemide 40 mg/d PO
    doses can be doubled if no response after 7 days
intraperitoneal therapy
    instillation of sclerosant e.g. bleomycin
    instill in 100-200 ml of fluid and posture patient
    predisposes to loculation
peritoneovenous shunts
    work poorly if fluid is bloody, viscous or loculated
    complications : fever, infection, shunt blockage, coagulopathy
    no evidence that shunts promote dissemination of the disease

LIVER METASTASES

Clinical features. Most patients with hepatic metastases are symptomatic (Table 3.48). Examination usually shows some degree of hepatomegaly which may be tender or nodular. The diagnosis is made on the clinical features and abnormal liver function tests and confirmed on scanning. Biopsy is rarely required to differentiate metastatic disease from other pathology.

Table 3.48 Hepatic metastases

general
    anorexia, nausea, weight loss
pain
    diffuse discomfort or pain in region of liver
    acute severe localized pain due to small capsular tears or perimetastatic hemorrhage
    shoulder pain caused by diaphragmatic irritation
marked hepatomegaly
    abdominal distension ± jaundice
    gastric compression and gastroesophageal reflux
    right lower lobe collapse ± small effusion

Treatment

The treatment options for hepatic metastases are listed in Table 3.49.

Table 3.49 Liver metastases in patients with advanced cancer : treatment options

systemic therapy	chemotherapy, hormonal (sensitive tumors)
surgery	excision, cryosurgery, injection
radiotherapy	external, internal (radioisotopes)
symptomatic	analgesics, antiemetics, dietary manipulation, corticosteroids

Surgery. Surgical resection of liver metastases may be of benefit for a single or small number of lesions but has no role in patients with widespread disease. Intraoperative or percutaneous cryotherapy is reported to be of benefit in selected patients; complications may be severe and the role of this technique is not defined. Intralesional injection of absolute alcohol has been used for small primary tumors; its role in the treatment of metastatic disease is not defined.

Radiotherapy. Doses of 24Gy in 3Gy fractions will produce significant symptomatic improvement in the majority of patients, with tolerable toxicity. Anorexia, nausea, vomiting and transient abnormalities of the liver function tests occur frequently. Higher doses of irradiation will cause radiation hepatitis with portal hypertension.

Symptomatic. Episodes of severe acute pain are treated with rest and opioid analgesics. Avoidance of fatty foods and the taking of multiple small meals can be of symptomatic benefit. Corticosteroids will improve symptoms in the majority of patients with hepatic metastases. Prednisolone 25-50mg/d usually produces a significant reduction in anorexia, nausea and discomfort. The dose may then be weaned to the minimum effective dose. The effect usually lasts for a number of weeks, following which further benefit can sometimes be gained by increasing the dose.

HEPATIC FAILURE AND ENCEPHALOPATHY

Cause. The causes of hepatic failure are listed in Table 3.50. Hepatic encephalopathy occurs in patients with impaired liver function, precipitated by a variety of factors (Table 3.51).

Table 3.50 Causes of hepatic failure

cancer : extensive hepatic replacement, biliary obstruction
drugs : anticancer, acetaminophen, antibiotics, others
radiation
alcohol
viral infection
systemic infection
hepatic vein occlusion, thrombosis (Budd-Chiari syndrome)
pericardial effusion, constriction

Table 3.51 Precipitating factors which may induce hepatic encephalopathy

increased production and absorption of ammonia and nitrogenous compounds	excess dietary protein gastrointestinal bleeding, constipation
hypovolemia	diuretics, hemorrhage, septicemia, rapid paracentesis
further liver damage	drug reactions, alcohol, viral hepatitis, septicemia
metabolic disturbance	uremia
drugs causing CNS depression	sedatives, tranquillizers, opioid analgesics

Clinical features. The clinical features of hepatic failure include jaundice, ascites, peripheral edema, hepatic encephalopathy and renal failure. Hepatic encephalopathy occurs when substances from the intestine reach the brain by porto-systemic shunting, via collateral vessels. The clinical features of hepatic encephalopathy vary from a mild disturbance of mental function to coma. There may be a non-rhythmical flapping tremor (asterixis, liver flap) and sweetish musty breath (fetor hepaticus).

Treatment

The treatment of hepatic failure depends on the cause and the stage of the patient's disease and prognosis. In patients who are terminally ill, only measures directed at patient comfort should be considered. In patients not considered terminally ill, the underlying cause is treated as well as measures to treat or prevent hepatic encephalopathy. The treatment of hepatic encephalopathy involves the withdrawal or treatment of any precipitating cause, dietary protein restriction, and oral lactulose (30 ml, 8-hourly) or neomycin (1 g daily) to reduce ammonia production. Agitation is treated with diazepam or other benzodiazepine. Hallucinations and psychoses are treated with chlorpromazine or haloperidol.

BILIARY TRACT OBSTRUCTION

Clinical features. Biliary tract obstruction is characterized by jaundice, light colored stools, dark urine and pruritus. Pain occurs less frequently in malignant biliary obstruction than in obstruction due to cholelithiasis.

Assessment. Liver function tests show elevation of the bilirubin and alkaline phosphatase out of proportion to the elevation in the transaminases. Ultrasonography will confirm biliary obstruction in up to 90% of cases; CT scanning is more accurate in defining the site and cause. The obstruction can be accurately localized by either endoscopic retrograde cholangiopancreatography (ERCP) or percutaneous transhepatic cholangiography (PTHC).

Treatment

Management options are listed in Table 3.52. Surgery or the placement of stents allow drainage of bile salts into the bowel and will prevent malabsorption. The choice of procedure depends on the site of the obstruction. Stents or catheters may be complicated by ascending cholangitis and require regular replacement. Radiotherapy has a limited role in the treatment of biliary obstruction due to the risk of radiation hepatitis. Pruritus will be relieved if the obstruction is overcome or can be palliated with various medications (see Pruritus, Chapter 8). Corticosteroids are occasionally of benefit.

Table 3.52   Treatment options for malignant biliary obstruction

systemic anticancer therapy (sensitive tumors)
surgical bypass
endoscopic placement of stent, catheter
percutaneous transhepatic placement of stent, catheter
radiotherapy
symptomatic care
    treatment of pruritus
    corticosteroids

> *Treatment must be appropriate to the stage of the patient's disease and the prognosis*

Terminal care. The treatment of biliary obstruction in the last days or week of life is symptomatic. If there is doubt about a patient's life expectancy, then nonsurgical stenting can be considered, especially if there is severe pruritus unresponsive to other measures.

Further Reading - see page 111

4 Genitourinary

> hematuria
> frequency and urgency
> urinary incontinence
> hesitancy
> urinary tract obstruction
> urinary catheters
>
> urinary infection
> renal failure
> prostatitis, epididymo-orchitis
> vaginitis, vaginal discharge
> uterine bleeding

HEMATURIA

Cause (Table 4.1).

Table 4.1 Causes of hematuria

infection	cystitis, prostatitis, urethritis
	septicemia
malignancy	primary or secondary tumor
iatrogenic	nephrostomy, ureteric stenting, catheterization, embolization, cystitis due to radiation, cyclophosphamide
bleeding diathesis	anticoagulants, coagulation disorder, thrombocytopenia, primary fibrinolysis
renal disease	renal vein thrombosis, paraneoplastic glomerular lesions
urolithiasis	

Clinical features. Hematuria occurring at the beginning of the urinary stream usually indicates a urethral lesion. Hematuria at the end of the stream is caused by bladder neck or prostatic lesions. Hematuria occurring throughout the urinary stream is usually associated with lesions above the bladder neck. Hematuria due to a bleeding diathesis is usually accompanied by signs of abnormal bleeding at other sites, except for fibrinolysis associated with prostate cancer which causes severe hematuria without evidence of systemic bleeding.

Assessment. Urine microscopy is performed to confirm the presence of red blood cells and distinguish urinary discoloration due to other pigments (Table 4.2); confirmatory microscopy is not necessary in patients with obvious hemorrhage. Microscopy may demonstrate evidence of infection or the presence of malignant cells and phase contrast microscopy can distinguish between upper and lower urinary tract bleeding. Further investigations are performed as clinically indicated including cystoscopy, retrograde or intravenous pyelography and CT scanning.

Treatment

The treatment is that of the cause although in many cases the bleeding is mild and no specific therapy is needed.

Fibrinolysis. Pathological fibrinolysis is treated with aminocaproic acid (Table 4.3). Tranexamic acid should be avoided as it may lead to formation of firm clots which are difficult to remove.

Table 4.2   Urinary discoloration not due to hematuria

Pigment	Color	Condition
urobilinogen	orange	hemolysis
bile	brown	obstructive jaundice
hemoglobin	red/dark brown	hemolysis
methemoglobin	brown	hemolysis
myoglobin	red	rhabdomyolysis
porphyrins	dark red	porphyria
melanin	brown	melanoma
anthocyanin	red	excess beetroot, berries
carotene	orange	excess carotene-containing foods
anthraquinone	red	excess rhubarb
drug metabolites	red	rifampicin, phenothiazines, dilantin, anthracyclines, phenindione, anthracene laxatives, phenolphthalein

Severe hematuria. Major hematuria demands intervention (Table 4.3). A rigid catheter is preferred as it allows removal of clots by suction; cystoscopy is sometimes required. Intravesical alum is frequently effective in stopping bleeding and causes few side effects. Persistent tumor bleeding can be treated by various other means.

Terminal care. A conservative approach is adopted whenever possible. Bleeding causing ureteric colic or clot retention is managed by the simplest and least invasive procedures which effectively control the symptoms.

Table 4.3   Treatment options for severe hematuria

catheterization or cystoscopy for clot evacuation
continuous saline bladder washout to prevent clot formation
persistent lower tract bleeding
    instillation alum : 50 ml 1% solution for 1h q4-12h, or by continuous washout
persistent tumor bleeding
    cystoscopy for diathermy, laser therapy or endoscopic tumor resection
    external radiotherapy
persistent bleeding due to radiation or cyclophosphamide cystitis
    instillation of formalin (requires general anesthetic)
fibrinolysis
    aminocaproic acid 5 g in first hour, then 1 g/h until bleeding settles, PO or IV infusion
hemorrhage from malignant infiltration of kidney
    radiotherapy, embolization, surgery

FREQUENCY AND URGENCY

Cause (Table 4.4). Frequency in combination with large urine volumes or bladder abnormalities will cause urgency.

Assessment. Clinical assessment, urine examination and monitoring the volume of the urinary output will usually define the cause. Cystoscopy is rarely required.

Treatment

The underlying cause is treated where possible.

Drug therapy. A small proportion of patients, including those with chronic bladder damage and those with neurological lesions, suffer persistent and troublesome frequency. Drug treatment which may be of benefit includes antidepressants,

Table 4.4 Causes of frequency

polyuria	high fluid intake, diuretic therapy, diabetes mellitus, diabetes insipidus, hypercalcemia
inflammation	infection: cystitis, prostatitis, urethritis chemotherapy, radiotherapy foreign bodies: stents, calculi
diminished bladder capacity	tumor, including extrinsic compression surgery post radiation, chemotherapy
detrusor instability/hyperactivity	neurological: CNS, spinal , pelvic nerve lesions infection anxiety
lower urinary tract obstruction	tumor, strictures, prostatomegaly, fecal impaction

anticholinergics and the combined anticholinergic smooth muscle relaxant, oxybutynin (Table 4.5). Calcium channel blockers or NSAIDs may also be of benefit. In the terminal care setting scopolamine hydrobromide can be given by subcutaneous infusion.

Table 4.5 Examples of bladder relaxant medications

antidepressant	imipramine	25-50 mg PO nocte
anticholinergic	propantheline	15-30 mg PO q6-12h
	scopolamine hydrobromide	0.6-1.2 mg/24h SC infusion
combined smooth muscle relaxant/anticholinergic	oxybutynin	2.5-5 mg PO q6-8h

URINARY INCONTINENCE

Cause (Table 4.6).

Table 4.6 Causes of urinary incontinence

overflow incontinence	
bladder outlet obstruction	malignant infiltration, prostatic enlargement fecal impaction, strictures, calculi
detrusor failure	anticholinergic drugs, anticholinergic side effects CNS, spinal cord or sacral nerve root lesions somnolence, confusion, dementia general weakness and debility
stress incontinence	
sphincter insufficiency	spinal cord or sacral nerve root lesions pelvic, urologic surgery malignant infiltration multiparity (prolapse), postmenopausal
urge incontinence	
detrusor hyperactivity or instability	polyuria, infection, inflammation malignant infiltration post radiation, chemotherapy CNS, spinal cord or sacral nerve root lesions anxiety
continuous incontinence	
fistulas	infiltration, radiotherapy, surgery

Assessment. Clinical assessment and urinalysis will usually indicate the cause. Patients with overflow incontinence complain of suprapubic pain, urgency and the frequent passage of small amounts of urine; the post-voiding residual volume is high. Stress incontinence leads to voiding when the patient coughs or lifts and strains. The post-voiding residual urine volume is low in patients with stress and urge incontinence. A ureterovaginal or vesicovaginal fistula will cause persistent dribbling of urine and can be demonstrated by instillation of methylene blue into the bladder.

Treatment

Treatment depends on the type of incontinence and the cause (Table 4.7).

Table 4.7 Incontinence : treatment options

bladder outlet obstruction
    relief of obstruction : surgery, radiotherapy, relief of fecal impaction
    stop drugs causing sedation or anticholinergic effects
    regular voiding, management of fluids
    α-blocker   : prazosin 0.5-1 mg PO q12h

detrusor failure
    stop drugs causing sedation or anticholinergic effects
    α-blocker   : prazosin 0.5-1 mg PO q12h
    cholinergic   : bethanechol 5-30 mg PO q6h

stress incontinence
    regular voiding, management of fluids
    pelvic muscle exercises, estrogens, pessaries, condom drainage
    adrenergic   : ephedrine 25-50 mg PO q8h
    antidepressant : doxepin or imipramine 25-50 mg PO nocte

urge incontinence
    regular voiding, management of fluids
    bladder relaxant medication (see Table 4.5)

General measures. These include access to toilet facilities, as well as the ability to use them or the availability of another person to provide assistance. Regular voiding is encouraged and fluid loads are avoided, especially in the evening. Drugs which cause sedation are avoided. Perineal skin care is important.

Overflow incontinence. Treatment with an α-blocker such as prazosin will improve urinary flow and bladder emptying; the main side effect is postural hypotension.

Detrusor failure. Treatment with an α-blocker is frequently helpful. Cholinergic drugs will stimulate detrusor function but are rarely useful unless the bladder weakness is due to an anticholinergic drug which needs to be continued. Bethanechol cannot be used if there is outlet obstruction; other side effects include intestinal colic, sweating and bradycardia. Patients with detrusor failure due to spinal cord disease, but with intact sacral reflexes, can be taught to void by reflex stimulation of the lower abdomen or perineum.

Stress incontinence. Exercises to strengthen pelvic musculature and treatment with estrogens can reduce incontinence in postmenopausal women. Women with pelvic prolapse may be helped by the insertion of a pessary. Condom drainage can be considered for men. Sphincter tone can be increased by adrenergic drugs but troublesome side effects limit the usefulness of these drugs. An antidepressant will help some patients.

Fistulas. Regular voiding may be of assistance as the amount of drainage from fistulas is less if the bladder is empty. For patients with a longer life expectancy, urinary diversion by either ureteric surgery or percutaneous nephrostomy can be considered. For patients with a shorter life expectancy, management is by catheterization which will reduce urine leakage through the fistula although incontinence pads and special attention to perineal skin care are still necessary.

Terminal care. The treatment of urinary incontinence is by catheterization.

HESITANCY

Cause. Urinary hesitancy, an abnormal delay between attempting to void and the start of micturition, is caused by bladder outflow obstruction or detrusor weakness (Table 4.6). The cause is usually clinically evident.

Treatment. Where possible and appropriate, the specific cause is treated. When hesitancy is due to the side effects of drugs given for other reasons, the doses are modified if possible. Bethanechol (5-30 mg PO q6h) helps some patients but side effects may be troublesome. Prazosin (0.5-1 mg PO q12h) may also be of benefit but causes postural hypotension. For patients too weak to sit or stand, nursing assistance to a more suitable position may help, but catheterization is often necessary.

URINARY TRACT OBSTRUCTION

Cause (Table 4.8). Cancers of the kidney, renal pelvis and ureter will cause unilateral obstruction. Cancers in the pelvis or retroperitoneal lymphadenopathy may cause unilateral or bilateral ureteric obstruction.

Table 4.8 Causes of urinary tract obstruction

upper tract (renal pelvis, ureter)	**lower tract** (bladder, urethra)
infiltration or compression by tumor	infiltration or compression by tumor
stricture : surgery, radiotherapy	benign enlargement of prostate
calculi	blood clots
blood clots	calculi
retroperitoneal fibrosis	infection
idiopathic or drug induced	urethral stricture
	fecal impaction
	detrusor failure
	anticholinergic side effects of drugs
	neurogenic

Assessment. Lower urinary tract obstruction usually presents as retention. The diagnosis of upper urinary tract obstruction is made on ultrasound or CT scanning; if doubt remains, retrograde pyelography can be considered.

Treatment

Lower tract obstruction. Lower urinary tract obstruction usually requires catheterization, at least temporarily. Treatment of obstructing tumor may involve surgery, radiotherapy, endoscopic resection or laser therapy. Other causes are treated appropriately.

Upper tract obstruction. Treatment is by cystoscopy and retrograde ureteric stenting or by a percutaneous nephrostomy inserted under radiological control. Antegrade ureteric stenting via the nephrostomy can be attempted several days later when local bleeding and swelling have settled. If successful, this will allow closure of the percutaneous nephrostomy. If ureteric stenting cannot be achieved, usually due to destruction of the ureteric orifices by carcinoma of the bladder, the nephrostomy is left in place permanently or some form of surgical urinary diversion considered. Ureteric stents may occlude, in which situation a cystogram will fail to show reflux of dye up the stent. Ureteric stents are routinely changed each 3 to 6 months.

Bilateral ureteric obstruction (or unilateral obstruction in a patient with a single functioning kidney) requires urgent intervention if renal function is to be preserved. However, careful consideration of the stage of the patient's disease and prognosis is required before embarking on therapy. For patients with advanced disseminated disease and no effective anticancer treatment available, allowing them to die with progressive uremia, without submitting them to invasive procedures, may be the less distressing course.

Post-obstruction diuresis. Relief of urinary obstruction frequently causes a post-obstruction diuresis requiring careful replacement therapy.

Terminal care. Lower urinary tract obstruction is relieved by catheterization; other investigations or therapy are inappropriate. In the last week or days of life, upper urinary tract obstruction with renal impairment should be managed symptomatically.

URINARY CATHETERS

Indications. The indications for long term catheterization are listed in Table 4.9.

Table 4.9 Indications for long term urinary catheterization

atonic bladder
persistent obstruction
persistent incontinence
management of decubitus or perineal ulceration or infection complicated by incontinence
to avoid painful movement required to change clothes and bed linen
patient comfort (terminally ill patients)

Infection. Regular irrigation delays the development of obstruction but increases the risk of infection. Prophylactic antibiotics do not prevent bacteriuria or reduce the incidence of urinary infections. Antibiotics should be considered if there are clinical signs of infection or repeated catheter blockages. Asymptomatic bacteriuria does not warrant treatment except for urease-producing organisms (most commonly *Proteus mirabilis*) which greatly increase the risk of calculus formation. A urinary antiseptic, hexamine hippurate, should be considered for patients with long term indwelling catheters; it requires urinary acidification to be effective.

Bypassing. Bypassing may be due to catheter obstruction or irritation of the bladder by the catheter. Obstruction is treated by flushing the catheter clear or by replacing it. For patients with a small or contracted bladder, the catheter balloon is inflated to only 5-10 ml (rather than the maximum volume written on the catheter) to avoid detrusor stimulation. Catheter bypassing is not treated by inserting a larger catheter which may cause more irritation. Some patients will benefit from the use of antispasmodic and bladder relaxant drugs (see Table 4.5)

Suprapubic catheters. A suprapubic urinary catheter is used if urethral catheterization is not possible and if catheterization is necessary during the course of pelvic radiotherapy. The principles of catheter care are the same. The advantages of a suprapubic catheter include greater patient comfort, fewer infections (prostatitis, epididymitis), avoidance of urethral strictures and ease with which the patient can be given a trial of voiding by clamping the tube intermittently.

URINARY INFECTION

Cause. Patients with advanced cancer are prone to urinary infection (Table 4.10).

Table 4.10 Predisposition to urinary infection in patients with cancer

general	immunosuppression : cancer, therapy general debility
obstruction, stasis	malignant infiltration, compression neurogenic bladder
tissue damage	cystitis : radiotherapy, chemotherapy surgery
iatrogenic fistulas	catheters, ureteric stents, nephrostomy tubes

Assessment. The diagnosis is established by the appropriate microbiological tests. The differential diagnosis includes non-infective causes of dysuria, as may result from the passage of urine over any inflamed mucosa.

Treatment

Treatment of urinary infection includes appropriate antibiotics, correction of predisposing factors, analgesia, urinary alkalinizing agents and encouragement regarding fluid intake. Treatment of obstruction should be considered, if possible, as urinary infection is difficult to eradicate if obstruction persists. Asymptomatic bacteriuria usually warrants no therapy except for urease-producing organisms such as *Proteus mirabilis* which predispose to calculus formation or if there are repeated catheter blockages.

RENAL FAILURE

Cause (Table 4.11). Renal tubular cell damage caused by radiological contrast media is more likely to occur in dehydrated patients and those with pre-existing renal impairment, diabetes mellitus and myeloma. Renal damage by drugs is more likely in patients who are elderly or dehydrated, those with pre-existing renal impairment or if two or more of the drugs are used at the same time.

Treatment

The treatment of renal failure depends on the cause, the degree of impairment and on the stage of the patient's disease. If impairment is mild, no further treatment may be necessary although other nephrotoxic influences need to be avoided. Patients for whom other anticancer therapy is available and those whose life expectancy is longer (except for renal failure) may appropriately be managed by dialysis. Other patients with advanced cancer, for whom further anticancer therapy is not available and whose life expectancy is limited, may best be treated without dialysis.

Table 4.11   Causes of renal impairment in patients with cancer

pre-renal
  inadequate fluid intake
  vomiting, diarrhea, gastrointestinal fistulas
  polyuria : hypercalcemia, diabetes insipidus and mellitus, diuretic therapy
  hemorrhage
  sepsis and shock
  liver disease (hepatorenal syndrome)
  third space fluid accumulation : ascites, bowel obstruction, vena caval obstruction
  pericardial tamponade, cardiac failure

renal
  tumor infiltration
  tumor-associated glomerular disease
  metabolic : hypercalcemia, hyperuricemia, lysozymuria, tumor lysis syndrome
  hyperviscosity : paraproteinemia, polycythemia, hyperleukocytosis
  amyloidosis
  disseminated intravascular coagulation (DIC)
  renal vein thrombosis
  radiation
  radiological contrast media
  drugs
      antitumor   : platinum, methotrexate, nitrosoureas, mitomycin
      antibiotics   : aminoglycosides, amphotericin, penicillins, cephalosporins
      other   : allopurinol, NSAIDs, cyclosporin
  pyelonephritis

post-renal   (see Urinary Tract Obstruction)

Terminal care. The development of oliguria or anuria during the last days of life requires no investigation or therapy unless it is associated with pain or increased dyspnea.

PROSTATITIS, EPIDIDYMO-ORCHITIS

Prostatitis and epididymo-orchitis usually occur after catheterization, endoscopy or following pelvic irradiation. The patient complains of dysuria associated with pain in the lower back and perineum and is febrile. The prostate gland is swollen and very tender. If there is also epididymo-orchitis, there will be pain and tender swelling of the epididymis and testicle. The responsible organism can usually be identified by urine examination, the most frequent being *E. coli*. Treatment is with appropriate antibiotics.

VAGINITIS, VAGINAL DISCHARGE

Cause. Patients with cancer are prone to develop vaginal infection for a variety of reasons including the frequent use of antibiotics and corticosteroids (Table 4.12).

Treatment. Management options are outlined in Table 4.12. Whatever the cause, secondary infection is common and is treated with appropriate antimicrobial therapy and attention to local hygiene. Metronidazole suppositories may reduce odor associated with vaginitis secondary to tumor infiltration, fistulas or radionecrosis.

Table 4.12 Vaginitis

infection	appropriate antimicrobial therapy
	attention to local hygiene
chemotherapy	treat secondary infection
radiation	acute : treat secondary infection
	chronic : topical estrogens
tumor	diathermy, laser, radiotherapy, surgery
	treat secondary infection
	metronidazole suppositories (for odor)
fistulas	rectovaginal : colostomy
	vesicovaginal : urinary diversion

ABNORMAL UTERINE BLEEDING

Cause (Table 4.13).

Table 4.13 Abnormalities of uterine bleeding

menorrhagia (heavy periods occurring regularly)
    idiopathic, dysfunctional
    uterine fibroid, IUD
    bleeding diathesis
irregular heavy bleeding
    anovulatory cycles
non-menstrual bleeding
    postcoital   : infection, polyp, tumor, bleeding diathesis
    intermenstrual   : progesterone-only pill, dysfunctional
    postmenopausal : cancer, radiation, infection, hormonal therapy, bleeding diathesis
amenorrhea
    hysterectomy
    estrogen deficiency : oophorectomy, chemotherapy, radiotherapy
    hormonal therapy   : tamoxifen, progestogens

Treatment. The treatment of bleeding due to recurrent tumor may include surgery, radiotherapy or local treatment with diathermy or laser. Bleeding due to hormonal therapy requires reassurance, although an assessment needs to be made to exclude cervical and uterine pathology. Except for women with hormone sensitive tumors, amenorrhea due to ovarian failure or oophorectomy is treated with hormone replacement therapy

Further Reading - see page 111

5 Cardiovascular

myocardial disease	edema
acute pericarditis	superior vena caval obstruction
pericardial effusion	inferior vena caval obstruction
constrictive pericarditis	lymphedema

MYOCARDIAL DISEASE

Cardiomyopathy causing cardiac failure can occur after anthracycline therapy; it is dose-dependent and should be avoidable. Treatment with an angiotensin converting enzyme inhibitor (ACE inhibitor) leads to improvement for most patients; traditional therapy with digoxin, diuretics and vasodilators was often ineffective.

ACUTE PERICARDITIS

Acute pericarditis due to irradiation occurs during or up to a few months after treatment. The patient complains of anterior chest pain and a pericardial rub is heard on examination. Clinically mild pericarditis can be managed by careful observation and treatment with a corticosteroid or NSAID. If there is evidence of significant effusion on echocardiography, pericardiocentesis should be considered.

PERICARDIAL EFFUSION

Cause (Table 5.1). Pericardial effusion is usually due to malignant infiltration but can also occur due to lymphatic obstruction in the mediastinum. Radiotherapy may cause pericardial effusion either as an acute (weeks/months) or late (years) side effect; the latter is often accompanied by signs of constrictive pericarditis.

Clinical features. The clinical features depend on the volume of pericardial fluid, the rate of accumulation and the underlying cardiac function. The pericardium normally contains less than 50 ml of fluid, but may accommodate several hundred milliliters if the accumulation is slow. If the increase is rapid, serious symptoms and signs will develop with small changes in the pericardial fluid volume. Pericardial tamponade exists when the amount of fluid present is sufficient to cause significant impairment of cardiac function.

Table 5.1 Pericardial disease

effusion
    malignant infiltration
    mediastinal lymphatic obstruction
    radiation
        acute pericarditis
        late pericardial effusion ± constriction
    uremia
    infection
constriction
    malignant encasement
    radiation

Patients present with dyspnea and may also have orthopnea and cough. On examination, the patient is anxious, sitting upright and leaning forward. There is a tachycardia, reduced systolic blood pressure and raised venous pressure. Pulsus paradoxus, the reduction of the pulse volume or a fall in the systolic blood pressure of more than 10 mm Hg occurring during inspiration, is present. The heart sounds may be distant or soft and there may be a pericardial rub. Pleural effusions, hepatomegaly and peripheral edema occur frequently.

Assessment. A chest x-ray may show enlargement of the cardiac shadow, which classically takes on a globular or boot shaped appearance. A normal cardiac shadow does not exclude tamponade, especially in patients who have had previous radiotherapy. Echocardiography will confirm the presence of an effusion, define its position and distribution and provide an assessment of cardiac function. An electrocardiogram (ECG) frequently shows non-specific changes. A CT scan will document the presence of an effusion but does not assess the effect on cardiac function.

Treatment

Pericardiocentesis. A pericardiocentesis is performed to relieve the hemodynamic abnormalities and to obtain fluid for diagnostic examination. This is performed under local anesthetic by percutaneous needle aspiration (by an experienced operator, with ECG control) or by a small subxiphoid incision. A drain tube can be inserted to allow further drainage or for subsequent instillation therapy. Failure of pericardiocentesis to relieve the signs of cardiac compression indicates that coexistent constriction is present, due either to radiation fibrosis or neoplastic encasement.

Further therapy for malignant infiltration (Table 5.2). Patients with malignant infiltration have been treated by instillation of various sclerosing agents although the use of these drugs is not of proven extra benefit; the most frequently used drug in the past, tetracycline, is no longer available. If the subxiphoid approach is used for initial pericardiocentesis, a pericardial window or opening in the parietal pericardium can be surgically created which will allow fluid to drain into the pericardiac tissues. Alternatively, a pericardial window can be created at thoracoscopy which allows drainage of fluid into the left pleural space. Patients with a shorter life expectancy can be considered for radiotherapy to the pericardium.

Table 5.2 Pericardial effusion : treatment options

pericardiocentesis
    to correct hemodynamic abnormalities
    to obtain fluid for diagnostic examination
malignant infiltration
    instillation of sclerosant
    systemic therapy (sensitive tumors)
    pericardial window
    radiation
radiation-induced
    early : observe, NSAID
    late : no treatment unless constriction also present
other causes (e.g. uremia, infection)
    appropriate therapy

CONSTRICTIVE PERICARDITIS

Cause. Constrictive pericardial disease in patients with cancer is due to either radiation fibrosis or neoplastic encasement.

Clinical features. Patients may complain of dyspnea and cough. Examination shows elevated venous pressure, a small pulse volume and lowering of the systolic blood pressure. Pulsus paradoxus is usually absent. Pleural effusions, hepatomegaly, ascites and dependent edema are common.

Assessment. The diagnosis is usually established by echocardiography but sometimes requires cardiac catheterization.

Treatment (Table 5.3). Patients with constrictive pericarditis due to radiotherapy can be considered for pericardiectomy. For patients with malignant encasement, pericardiectomy is frequently not feasible; pericardial irradiation can be considered.

Table 5.3 Pericardial constriction : treatment options

radiotherapy fibrosis	pericardiectomy
tumor encasement	systemic therapy (sensitive tumors)
	radiotherapy
	pericardiectomy

EDEMA

Cause (Table 5.4).

Edema associated with raised capillary venous pressure. The edema is peripheral and dependent and is more marked in the evening. Examination shows raised jugular venous pressure without postural hypotension. Management of the edema involves salt restriction and diuretics. Digoxin, vasodilators and angiotensin converting enzyme inhibitors (ACE inhibitors) can be considered for cardiac failure.

Edema associated with reduced capillary oncotic pressure. The edema is generalized, may be most noticeable in the face and is more marked in the morning. Examination often shows postural hypotension without elevation of the venous pressure. The treatment is that of the cause and infusions of protein or albumin give slight or no relief. Dietary sodium restriction and diuretic therapy, particularly with spironolactone, may be of benefit.

Table 5.4 Causes of edema

localized
    venous or lymphatic obstruction
    immobility, immobilization
generalized
    raised capillary venous pressure
        heart failure
        venous obstruction
        (iatrogenic) fluid overload
    decreased capillary oncotic pressure (hypoproteinemia)
        poor dietary intake, malabsorption
        liver disease
        repeated aspiration of effusions
        catabolic state associated with cancer
        nephrotic syndrome

SUPERIOR VENA CAVAL OBSTRUCTION

Cause. Superior vena caval (SVC) obstruction is usually due to compression or invasion by tumor. Less commonly, thrombosis occurs secondary to a centrally placed catheter.

Clinical features. The patient is dyspneic and appears cyanosed. There is edema of the face, neck and upper limbs. The neck veins are distended and there are dilated veins on the backs of the hands which do not collapse when the arm is elevated. There may be other symptoms related to mediastinal disease including cough, dysphagia, chest pain or hoarseness. Neurological symptoms include headache, dizziness, blurred vision and syncope, all of which are aggravated or precipitated by leaning forward or stooping. The diagnosis can be made on clinical grounds and chest x-ray or CT scanning will usually show mediastinal tumor.

Treatment

General measures. Dexamethasone (16-24 mg/d) is of benefit to some patients. Other general symptomatic measures include bed rest with the head elevated, oxygen administration, fluid and salt restriction and diuretic therapy in moderate to high dose.

Treatment of tumor. Small cell lung cancer or lymphoma can be treated with either radiotherapy or chemotherapy, depending on what previous treatment has been given. Patients with other tumors are treated with radiotherapy. Recurrent and refractory obstruction can be treated with angioplasty and stenting.

Catheter-associated thrombosis. Patients with catheter-associated thrombosis are treated with heparin and the catheter removed. Some patients with catheter-associated thrombosis have been successfully treated with fibrinolytic therapy.

INFERIOR VENA CAVAL OBSTRUCTION

Cause. The inferior vena cava (IVC) may be obstructed by compression, direct infiltration or thrombosis.

Clinical features. Lesser degrees of IVC obstruction often pass unnoticed except for some peripheral edema, due to the availability of collateral venous circulation. Complete IVC obstruction causes marked swelling of the lower limbs with pitting edema extending up to at least the level of the iliac crests and including the perineum and external genitalia. There is venous dilatation on the anterior abdominal wall and there may be ascites.

Treatment. IVC obstruction occurs most commonly in the terminal phase and treatment is symptomatic. IVC thrombosis in a patient with apparently longer life expectancy may be treated with anticoagulation.

LYMPHEDEMA

Cause. Lymphedema is caused by obstruction or interruption of the lymphatic system by surgery, radiotherapy or tumor. It develops most frequently after surgical lymphadenectomy or radiotherapy to the inguinal region or axilla and the incidence is increased if both modalities of treatment are used. Limbs affected by lymphedema are particularly prone to cellulitis and each episode of infection can aggravate the degree of edema.

Clinical features. Lymphedema is non-pitting edema of the subcutaneous tissues that does not resolve with either rest or elevation. It is unsightly, uncomfortable and compromises function. In severe and chronic cases there is gross swelling associated with constant pain and a functionally useless limb.

Treatment

General measures. Strategies for the treatment of established lymphedema are listed in Table 5.5. There needs to be scrupulous care of the skin and nails as well as the avoidance of any injuries, however minor, which might lead to infection. If infection occurs it is treated promptly with antibiotics which often need to be continued for several weeks.

Table 5.5 Treatment of lymphedema
general skin and nail care
avoid trauma - protective garments, gloves
- no injections
- electric shaver
- insect repellents, sun blockout creams
prompt and adequate treatment of infection
support garments
exercise
massage
compression pumps
benzopyrone

Support garments. Patients are fitted with a well-fitting pressure sleeve or stocking. A support garment should feel comfortable and not tight - the aim is not to reduce limb volume but to prevent further fluid accumulation. Patients are encouraged to use the limb as normally as possible, as active movement may improve lymph drainage. The affected limb can be elevated when resting. Patients with leg edema should avoid prolonged periods of standing.

Massage. A program of daily massage will help many patients. Massage aims to stimulate lymphatics in the skin and facilitate opening of collateral channels. Massage is started on the trunk adjacent to the swollen limb, stroking the skin away from the limb; the process is continued progressively down the limb. The massage strokes should be firm enough to move the skin but not redden it. Support garments are worn between treatments.

Compression pumps. Compression pumps provide intermittent sequential pneumatic compression of the limb, repetitively massaging the limb in a central direction. Pumps need to be used daily or at least several times a week, indefinitely, with pressure support garments worn between treatments. Pumps cannot be used if there is evidence of infection or thrombosis of the affected limb. Pumps will prevent progression or produce gradual improvement for some patients.

Benzopyrone. Treatment with oral benzopyrone is reported to be useful in reducing lymphedema but requires many months to be effective and may not add significantly to standard therapy outlined above.

Surgery. A variety of surgical procedures have been advocated for the treatment of lymphedema, none of which are effective.

Further Reading - see page 111

6 Hematological

> anemia
> polycythemia
> leukocyte disorders
> platelet disorders
>
> thrombosis
> bleeding
> hyperviscosity

ANEMIA

Cause (Table 6.1). Anemia is frequently multifactorial in patients with cancer.

Table 6.1 Classification of anemia

decreased red cell production	increased red cell destruction
anemia of chronic disease	hemolytic anemia
chemotherapy, radiotherapy	infection
marrow infiltration	hypersplenism
iron deficiency	increased plasma volume (spurious anemia)
megaloblastic anemia	paraproteinemia
myelodysplasia	inappropriate ADH
red blood cell loss	
bleeding	

Assessment and Treatment

If the anemia is mild or the cause obvious, further investigation is often unnecessary. If the anemia is severe, an attempt should be made to define the cause.

Anemia of chronic disease. This is the most common type of anemia in patients with cancer. It is usually a diagnosis of exclusion, no other cause for anemia being found. There is a normochromic normocytic anemia; the serum iron and iron binding capacity are reduced and the serum ferritin level is normal or increased. The anemia is rarely severe and the treatment is that of the underlying disease. Hematinic therapy with iron, vitamin B_{12} or folate is ineffective. Transfusion may provide temporary symptomatic improvement.

Marrow infiltration. Marrow infiltration produces a leukoerythroblastic blood film with immature white cells, nucleated red cells and marked variation in the size and shape of the red cells (anisopoikilocytosis). Treatment is that of the underlying condition.

Chemotherapy, radiotherapy. Chemotherapy or radiotherapy produces pancytopenia with reduction of the white cell and platelet counts as well as anemia. The changes usually resolve spontaneously and transfusion can be given if required for symptoms.

Iron deficiency. Iron deficiency and bleeding produce a hypochromic microcytic anemia. The serum iron and ferritin are reduced, the iron binding capacity elevated. Treatment is with replacement therapy and by treatment of the cause of bleeding. Oral or parenteral iron or transfusion can be given, depending on the severity and speed of onset of the anemia.

Megaloblastic anemia. Vitamin B_{12} or folate deficiency produce a macrocytic anemia with megaloblastic changes in the marrow. Measurement of the serum vitamin B_{12} and folate levels will document deficiency and treatment is with appropriate replacement therapy.

Microangiopathic hemolytic anemia. This is associated with disseminated mucin-secreting adenocarcinomas. Investigation shows hemolytic anemia with microangiopathic red cell changes (fragmentation, shistocytes). It is usually associated with disseminated intravascular coagulation and thrombocytopenia. Treatment is usually unsuccessful unless there is effective therapy for the underlying malignancy.

Transfusion. Decisions regarding blood transfusions for patients with advanced cancer depend on the stage of the disease and life expectancy as well as the speed of onset and severity of the symptoms of anemia. Acute anemia due to blood loss or serious infection usually requires transfusion. Recommendations regarding transfusion for patients with chronic anemia are summarized in Table 6.2.

Table 6.2 Indications for blood transfusion

acute anemia			
chronic anemia:	Hb < 8-9 g/dl	and	symptomatic
	Hb 8-9 g/dl	and	continued or likely hemorrhage
			planned surgery
			planned radiotherapy
			planned chemotherapy
			serious infection
			doubt as to whether transfusion would be of symptomatic benefit
			unexplained weakness, fatigue or dyspnea
	Hb > 9-10 g/dl	and	symptomatic (as a result of cardiac or respiratory insufficiency)

Erythropoietin. Treatment of patients with cancer and anemia with recombinant human erythropoietin (EPO) leads to a significant rise in hemoglobin and reduction in transfusion requirement. It is administered by injection three times weekly and is well tolerated. However, it is very expensive and its role in routine oncology practice remains to be defined.

POLYCYTHEMIA (ERYTHROCYTOSIS)

Polycythemia is defined as elevation of the hemoglobin or hematocrit (packed cell volume, PCV) above the upper limit of the normal range.

Cause (Table 6.3). In spurious or relative polycythemia the elevated hematocrit is due to contraction of the plasma volume.

Table 6.3 Causes of polycythemia

true or absolute polycythemia
    primary : polycythemia rubra vera
    secondary
        hypoxia: lung disease, high altitude
        increased erythropoietin : renal disease, certain uncommon tumors, androgen therapy
spurious or relative polycythemia
    reduced plasma volume : dehydration, diuretic therapy

Treatment

Polycythemia vera. Polycythemia vera requires treatment to reduce the risk of thrombosis and hemorrhage and to prevent the complications of hyperviscosity. Venesection or phlebotomy alone may be adequate if the abnormalities are mild but myelosuppressive treatment with cytotoxic therapy or radioactive phosphorus (^{32}P) are frequently required. The aim is to keep the hematocrit at or near the upper limit of normal, especially if surgery is planned.

Secondary polycythemia. Patients with polycythemia secondary to hypoxia rarely require therapy. Despite marked elevation of the hematocrit, the patient is asymptomatic and there is no major risk of bleeding or thrombosis. Patients with severe symptoms of hyperviscosity or right heart failure may benefit from cautious venesection. The treatment of other secondary polycythemias is directed at the cause.

LEUKOCYTE DISORDERS

Leukocytosis

The common causes of leukocytosis are shown in Table 6.4. Recognition of these may spare patients unnecessary investigations or empiric treatment for suspected infections. If required, the treatment of leukocytosis is that of the underlying cause.

Table 6.4 Causes of leukocytosis

myeloid leukocytosis	
predominantly mature neutrophils	
solid tumors	post-splenectomy
myeloproliferative disorders	inflammation and tissue necrosis
chemotherapy-recovery phase	infection
colony stimulating factor therapy	hemorrhage
corticosteroids	hemolysis
leukemoid (with circulating immature leukocytes)	
myeloid leukemia	chemotherapy-recovery phase
myeloproliferative disorders	infection
marrow infiltration	inflammation
eosinophilia	
lymphoproliferative disorders	allergic disorders
myeloproliferative disorders	dermatitis
solid tumors	parasitic infection
basophilia	
myeloproliferative disorders	
monocytosis	
solid tumors	infection
lymphoproliferative disorders	inflammation
myeloproliferative disorders	collagen diseases
monocytic leukemia	
lymphocytosis	
lymphatic leukemia	infection
lymphoma	drugs
solid tumors	

Hyperleukocytosis. Hyperviscosity may occur with myeloid leukemias if the white cell count is >100,000 x 10^9/l Treatment needs to be initiated before irreversible cerebral or pulmonary damage occurs (see Hyperviscosity).

Sweet's syndrome. This is the association of neutrophilia, pyrexia, painful cutaneous plaques and arthralgia occurring in patients with cancer. The treatment is that of the underlying disease; there may be symptomatic improvement with corticosteroids.

Leukopenia

Lymphopenia. Lymphopenia occurs frequently as a result of chemotherapy, radiotherapy or treatment with corticosteroids. It requires no investigation or treatment.

Neutropenia. Causes of neutropenia are listed in Table 6.5. Neutropenia predisposes to infection, the risk being proportional to the severity and duration. Neutropenia also causes mucositis, especially involving the gastrointestinal tract. Treatment-related neutropenia usually resolves spontaneously; in other situations, treatment should be directed at the underlying cause.

Table 6.5 Causes of neutropenia

cancer treatment	chemotherapy, radiotherapy
marrow infiltration	
megaloblastosis	vitamin B_{12}, folic acid deficiency
infection	
hypersplenism	
drug-induced	antibiotics, NSAIDs, phenothiazines, anticonvulsants, diuretics, oral hypoglycemics, antidepressants, anxiolytics

PLATELET DISORDERS

Thrombocytosis (Platelets > 400,000 x 10^9/l)

Cause (Table 6.6).

Table 6.6 Causes of thrombocytosis

chronic myeloproliferative disorders : ET, PRV, CML
other cancers : solid tumors, lymphomas
hemorrhage
postoperative
splenectomy
chemotherapy : recovery phase
other : infection, inflammation, hemolysis, vincristine therapy

Myeloproliferative disorders. Marked elevation of the platelet count (over 800-1000 x 10^9/l) occurs in the chronic myeloproliferative disorders — essential thrombocythemia (ET), polycythemia vera (PRV) and chronic myeloid leukemia (CML). It predisposes to both thrombosis and hemorrhage. Treatment is by myelosuppressive therapy with either cytotoxic drugs or radioactive phosphorus (^{32}P). Normalization of the count reduces the risk of thrombosis and hemorrhage to near normal. If surgery is planned, the count should be reduced to as near normal as possible preoperatively and care should be taken that postoperative anticoagulation is adequate.

Other causes. The thrombocytosis associated with other tumors and the other causes in Table 6.6 is usually mild (platelet count 400-800 x 10^9/l) and does not require specific treatment. Other factors predisposing to thrombosis need to be avoided or treated and care taken that postoperative anticoagulation is adequate.

Thrombocytopenia (Platelets <150,000 x 10^9/l)

Cause (Table 6.7).

Table 6.7 Causes of thrombocytopenia

diminished platelet production
    marrow infiltration : solid tumors, hematological malignancies
    cancer treatment : chemotherapy, radiotherapy
    drugs : thiazides, alcohol, estrogens, interferon
    vitamin B_{12} or folate deficiency
    viral infection
increased platelet destruction
    non-immune : infection
                disseminated intravascular coagulation (DIC)
                microangiopathic hemolytic anemia
                hypersplenism
    immune   : drugs
                lymphoproliferative disorders
                solid tumors
                idiopathic (ITP)

Assessment. Bone marrow examination should be considered for patients with a platelet count <70 x 10^9/l for which the cause is not apparent. This will distinguish impaired production from increased peripheral destruction and will demonstrate any marrow pathology.

Clinical features. The risk of bleeding depends on the degree of thrombocytopenia (Table 6.8) and will be greater if there is abnormal platelet function (see below).

Table 6.8 Thrombocytopenia and bleeding

Platelet count		
>50x10^9/l	-	easy bruising, spontaneous bleeding rare
20-50x10^9/l	-	excessive bruising, increased bleeding with trauma
<20x10^9/l	-	significant risk of spontaneous bleeding

Treatment. The treatment of thrombocytopenia depends on the cause and severity. Any drugs which might cause thrombocytopenia or diminished platelet function should be stopped if possible. If severe, platelet transfusions may be required.

Abnormal platelet function

Cause (Table 6.9).

Table 6.9 Abnormal platelet function

dyshemopoiesis	myeloid leukemia
	chronic myeloproliferative disorders
	myelodysplasia
uremia	
paraproteinemia	
drugs	aspirin, NSAIDs, penicillins

Clinical features. Abnormal platelet function can cause bleeding when the platelet count is normal or more severe bleeding than expected from the degree of thrombocytopenia.

Treatment. Drug-induced platelet dysfunction will resolve if the responsible drug is stopped. The intrinsic abnormalities in dyshemopoietic conditions are not correctable and platelet transfusions are required for significant bleeding. In the other situations, platelet function will improve with treatment of the underlying cause.

THROMBOSIS

Cause. Factors predisposing to thrombosis in patients with cancer are listed in Table 6.10. In addition, many patients are elderly.

Disseminated intravascular coagulation. There is evidence that many of the thrombotic events in patients with cancer are part of a hypercoagulable state related to disseminated intravascular coagulation (DIC). Sophisticated investigations show evidence of chronic DIC in as many as 75% of patients with malignant disease, with increased turnover or consumption of clotting factors, platelets and fibrinogen, associated with increased levels of fibrinolytic degradation products. Routine laboratory tests are often normal.

Table 6.10 Predisposition to thrombosis in malignant disease

vessel wall abnormalities
    malignant invasion
    ischemic damage, hypoxia
    corticosteroid therapy
reduced flow
    immobilization, bed rest
    malignant invasion, compression
    congestive heart failure, edematous states
    hyperviscosity syndromes
    intravascular catheters
platelet abnormalities
    thrombocytosis
    platelet activation by tumor cell products
coagulation factor abnormalities
    increased factor levels : estrogens
    increased levels of activated factors : tumor-associated procoagulants
    decreased hepatic clearance of activated factors : liver disease

Clinical features. The signs and symptoms of venous thrombosis are no different to those in patients without malignancy and the diagnosis is made in the same manner with venography, ultrasonography or venous pool scanning. Venous thromboses occurring in patients with chronic DIC are more likely to be recurrent or multiple. Trousseau's syndrome is recurrent superficial thrombophlebitis which is characteristically associated with intra-abdominal cancer.

Treatment

Decisions regarding anticoagulation for patients with advanced cancer need to be individualized, considering the potential benefits and risks of the treatment, and should be appropriate to the stage of the disease and prognosis (Table 6.11). Standard

Table 6.11 Contraindications to anticoagulant therapy

absolute	*relative*
significant active bleeding	recent bleeding
severe bleeding tendency	bleeding tendency
recent brain or spinal cord surgery	active peptic ulceration
	recent major surgery
	cerebral metastases
	uncontrolled hypertension
	severe renal failure
	severe hepatic failure
	terminally ill

treatment for venous thrombosis is anticoagulation with heparin and warfarin (Table 6.12). Surgical placement of vena caval filters may be of value in certain situations, and thrombolytic therapy may be considered in exceptional circumstances.

Heparin. Heparin is given by intravenous infusion or subcutaneous injection each 8-12 hours. Subcutaneous heparin is useful for patients requiring continued heparin therapy and those being treated at home. It is monitored in the same way as intravenous therapy. Continued treatment with heparin should be considered for patients with definite or presumptive evidence of underlying DIC, including those with recurrent thrombosis on warfarin therapy and multiple or arterial thromboses.

A number of low molecular weight heparin preparations are available which are effective in the prevention and treatment of venous thrombosis. They are administered subcutaneously, are associated with less hemorrhage, require less laboratory monitoring and are suitable for home treatment.

Table 6.12 Management of venous thrombosis

initial therapy
> heparin : 5-10 d IV; APTT : 1.5-2.5xN
> alternatives : vena caval filter (heparin contraindicated)
> > SC heparin (home care)
> > no anticoagulation (terminal care)

continuation therapy
> warfarin : 3-6 months PO; INR 2-3
> alternatives : no treatment (advanced malignant disease)
> > continued heparin (evidence of DIC)

recurrent thrombosis on warfarin
> INR subtherapeutic : heparin, then warfarin to INR of 2-3 or 3-4
> > alternatives : continued heparin (evidence of DIC)
> > > no treatment (advanced disease)
> > > vena caval filter
> INR therapeutic : heparin, then warfarin to INR of 3-4
> > alternatives : continued heparin
> > > vena caval filter
> > > no treatment (advanced disease)

recurrent thrombosis after completing warfarin therapy
> heparin, then warfarin to INR of 2-3
> alternatives : continued heparin (evidence of DIC)
> > no treatment (advanced disease)
> > vena caval filter

Warfarin. Patients with cancer receiving warfarin require more frequent laboratory monitoring than patients without malignant disease. Features commonly associated with advancing cancer, including poor nutritional intake and progressive liver dysfunction, will predispose to over-anticoagulation. Warfarin therapy may also be interfered with by other medications, a problem which is usually managed by instructing the patient to take the other medications in the same dose every day. This is often not feasible for the palliative care patient requiring repeated changes of drugs or doses, and frequent laboratory testing is necessary.

Surgical insertion of vena caval filter. A transvenously inserted Greenfield vena caval filter is the treatment of choice for preventing pulmonary embolism in patients for whom anticoagulant therapy is complicated or contraindicated. Vena cava filters are not of use if the thrombosis involves the vena cava itself or in patients with chronic DIC who develop thromboses at multiple sites.

Thrombolytic therapy. The thrombolytic agents urokinase and streptokinase convert plasminogen to plasmin, leading to rapid clot lysis, but there is a substantial risk of hemorrhage. The indications for thrombolytic therapy for patients with cancer are shown in Table 6.13; in most instances the risks outweigh the potential benefits. Intracranial disease is an absolute contraindication and patients should be scanned for occult cerebral metastases before starting treatment.

Table 6.13 Thrombolytic therapy in cancer patients

contraindications
intracranial pathology
recent (less than 10 days) surgery
active or recent bleeding
bleeding diathesis
presence of lesions prone to hemorrhage
indications
pulmonary embolism : massive embolism with cardiac decompensation, no contraindications and a reasonable life expectancy
venous catheter dysfunction

Thrombolytic therapy for central venous catheter blockage. Thrombolytic therapy is indicated for central venous catheter dysfunction caused by a thrombus at the tip of the catheter. Five thousand units of either streptokinase or urokinase are diluted to the volume which will just fill the occluded catheter, then instilled and left in place for one hour. This treatment is usually successful and can be repeated as often as necessary without risk of systemic bleeding.

Terminal care. Decisions regarding anticoagulation in terminally ill patients are difficult. Heparin will reduce pain and swelling in the leg and can hasten resolution of chest pain and dyspnea from pulmonary embolism. Whether heparin is employed depends on the severity of the symptoms and the patient's estimated life expectancy. Heparin therapy does not necessarily require hospitalization as heparin (or a low molecular weight heparin preparation) can be given by subcutaneous injection at home. Warfarin therapy is not indicated.

BLEEDING DISORDERS

Purpura

Purpura is defined as bleeding into the skin or mucous membranes.
Cause (Table 6.14).

Table 6.14 Causes of purpura

mechanical purpura	allergic purpura (Henoch-Schönlein)
orthostatic purpura	infection
purpura simplex ('easy bruising')	paraproteinemia
senile purpura	thrombocytopenia (see Table 6.7)
Cushing's syndrome, corticosteroids	abnormal platelet function (see Table 6.9)
vitamin C deficiency	coagulation abnormalities (see Table 6.15)
amyloidosis	

Clinical features. Mechanical purpura occurs at pressure areas or under adhesive bandages; paroxysmal coughing or violent retching can produce purpura over the head and neck as well as conjunctival hemorrhage. Orthostatic purpura is seen on the lower legs in edematous states. Purpura simplex or easy bruising consists of purpura or ecchymoses which develop in response to otherwise trivial trauma; it is common in women of reproductive age and requires no specific therapy. Senile purpura is the same as purpura simplex except that it occurs in older people and requires only reassurance. Patients with Cushing's syndrome or receiving corticosteroids develop a similar syndrome which is reversible if the drug is withdrawn. Amyloidosis can involve the cutaneous vessels and produce purpura which often affects the eyelids. In addition, any of the conditions which cause a generalized bleeding diathesis can cause purpura.

Coagulation Disorders

Cause (Table 6.15). Vitamin K and adequate liver function are necessary for the synthesis of most coagulation factors. Acute or subacute DIC occurs as a result of sepsis and shock or in association with mucin secreting adenocarcinomas and acute leukemia. Fibrinolysis occurs with streptokinase and urokinase and in patients with carcinoma of the prostate.

Table 6.15 Causes of generalized bleeding

thrombocytopenia	(see Table 6.7)
abnormal platelet function	(see Table 6.9)
coagulation abnormalities	
vitamin K deficiency	(see Table 6.16)
liver disease	
anticoagulation : heparin, warfarin	
coagulation factor inhibitors	
disseminated intravascular coagulation (DIC)	
fibrinolysis : pathological, therapeutic	

Assessment. The diagnosis of the cause of clinical bleeding is based on laboratory investigations.

Treatment. The treatment of vitamin K deficiency is that of the cause (Table 6.16) together with oral or parenteral supplements. Patients with active bleeding or severe hepatic dysfunction require transfusion of plasma. The treatment of acute or subacute DIC is with replacement of clotting factors and platelets and treatment of the underlying cause; the use of heparin is controversial. The initial treatment of fibrinolysis should be with clotting factor replacement; the fibrinolytic inhibitor aminocaproic acid can be used but may predispose to thromboses.

Table 6.16 Vitamin K deficiency

decreased intake
decreased production in small bowel
    small bowel disease, antibiotics
decreased absorption
    small bowel resection, bypass, disease (malabsorption)
    biliary obstruction (intrahepatic or extrahepatic)
    cholestyramine
decreased utilization
    liver disease, coumarin anticoagulants

Local bleeding

Cause. Troublesome local bleeding is usually related to recurrent tumor.

Topical therapy. A variety of agents can be applied topically to control local bleeding (Table 6.17).

Table 6.17 Treatment options for local bleeding

local therapy	*topical therapy*
radiotherapy	epinephrine (1:1000)
diathermy, laser, cryotherapy	thrombin
embolization	tranexamic acid : 500 mg tab dissolved in 5 ml
	aluminum astringents : 1% alum solution
systemic therapy	: sucralfate paste
correction of bleeding diathesis	hemostatic dressings : e.g. calcium alginate
tranexamic acid 1g PO q8h	silver nitrate sticks

Local therapy. Local radiotherapy is the standard treatment for local tumor-related bleeding which is not responding to topical therapy. In some situations, local tumor bleeding is amenable to diathermy, laser treatment or cryotherapy. Persistent local bleeding, such as that due to a carcinoma of the kidney, may be treated by embolization.

Systemic therapy. Any systemic bleeding diathesis is corrected. Oral tranexamic acid will improve bleeding for some patients; it is not recommended for patients with hematuria as it may cause clot formation.

HYPERVISCOSITY SYNDROME

The hyperviscosity syndrome occurs when the blood viscosity is increased sufficiently to cause interference with the microcirculation. Intravascular stasis in the capillary circulation leads to local hypoxia.

Cause. Hyperviscosity may be caused by excessive amounts of protein in paraproteinemia (multiple myeloma, Waldenstrom's macroglobulinemia), hyperleukocytosis in myeloid leukemia or erythrocytosis in polycythemia vera.

Clinical features (Table 6.18). Untreated, the hyperviscosity syndrome can cause irreversible damage to the brain, eyes, kidney and lung and can be fatal.

Treatment. Treatment comprises physical removal of the cause of the hyperviscosity as well as therapy for the underlying disorder : leukopheresis and chemotherapy for myeloid leukemia, venesection and myelosuppressive therapy for polycythemia vera, and plasmapheresis and chemotherapy for paraproteinemia. Blood transfusion must not be given until hyperviscosity is controlled.

Table 6.18 Clinical features of the hyperviscosity syndrome

bleeding	purpura and mucosal hemorrhage
neurological	headache, nausea, dizziness
	ataxia, dysarthria
	confusion, somnolence, coma, seizures
visual	blurred vision, diplopia, blindness
	distended retinal veins, hemorrhages, papilledema
cardiac	dyspnea, angina
	congestive heart failure
renal	renal impairment
pulmonary	cough, dyspnea
	respiratory impairment, adult respiratory distress syndrome

Further Reading - see page 111

7 Musculoskeletal

> muscle weakness   myoclonus
> muscle cramps   hypertrophic pulmonary osteoarthropathy
> muscle spasm   bone metastases

MUSCLE WEAKNESS

Causes (Table 7.1).

Table 7.1 Muscle weakness

central or peripheral nervous system disease or damage
metabolic
    hypercalcemia, hypokalemia, hypomagnesemia, hyperthyroidism
myopathic syndromes
    polymyositis, dermatomyositis
    myasthenic syndrome (Eaton-Lambert)
    corticosteroid myopathy : iatrogenic, ectopic ACTH

Myopathic syndromes

Polymyositis and dermatomyositis. These uncommon syndromes are often associated with malignant disease. The patient complains of muscle pain and tenderness and proximal muscular weakness develops over weeks or months. Dermatomyositis is distinguished by the presence of violet discoloration affecting the eyelids with blotch patches on the cheeks and nose and over the knuckles and elbows. Investigations show elevation of the ESR and CPK, a myopathic pattern on electromyographic (EMG) examination and inflammation and muscle fiber necrosis on biopsy. Control of the underlying tumor may lead to improvement. Treatment with corticosteroids and immunosuppression is of benefit in some cases.

Myasthenic (Eaton-Lambert) syndrome. This uncommon syndrome is usually associated with small cell carcinoma of the lung. It is caused by an antibody directed against the calcium channels in the presynaptic membrane of the neuromuscular junction, resulting in impaired release of acetylcholine. It is characterized by proximal muscle weakness which improves with exercise, distinguishing it from true myasthenia. Ptosis, diplopia, dysarthria and a variety of less common neurological abnormalities may occur. EMG examination shows characteristic abnormalities. The neurological symptoms may improve with successful control of the underlying malignancy. Anticholinesterase agents such as pyridostigmine lead to improvement in some cases, as may treatment with corticosteroids. Drugs which enhance acetylcholine release, diaminopyridine and guanidine, are also reported to be of benefit.

Corticosteroid myopathy. Patients treated with corticosteroids for more than a few weeks are at risk of developing proximal muscle weakness. The myopathy will improve within a few weeks of stopping corticosteroid therapy although this is frequently not feasible.

Patients with tumors secreting ectopic ACTH may also develop proximal myopathy. This may improve with successful control of the underlying tumor. If this is not possible, drugs that inhibit adrenal corticosteroid production, such as aminoglutethimide or metyrapone, can be used. These drugs produce adrenal suppression and patients require corticosteroid replacement at physiological dosage.

MUSCLE CRAMPS

Muscle cramps are acute painful muscular contractions.

Cause. Cramps occur in well people during or after strenuous exercise and at night, probably due to hyperexcitability of the intramuscular portion of the motor nerve. Cramps occur in patients with cancer for a variety of reasons (Table 7.2).

Tetany. Tetany is a cramp-like involuntary spasm usually involving distal muscles, as with carpopedal spasm. It occurs with hypocalcemia and hypomagnesemia but is most frequently seen in patients with anxiety who hyperventilate. Treatment is by correction of the metabolic abnormality or, in the case of hyperventilation, teaching breathing control and relaxation exercises.

Table 7.2 Causes of muscle cramps

idiopathic	
resting : post-exercise, nocturnal	
during exercise	
pathological	
neuromuscular	nerve root damage by tumor, radiotherapy
	paraneoplastic neuromyopathy
	peripheral neuropathy due to chemotherapy
	polymyositis, dermatomyositis
metabolic	dehydration, hypocalcemia, hypomagnesemia, uremia
	anxiety with hyperventilation
drugs	diuretics, medroxyprogesterone, aminoglutethimide, amphotericin, cimetidine

Treatment

A muscle cramp usually resolves with passive stretching of the muscle. Treatment of pathological muscle cramps includes the correction of metabolic abnormalities, withholding drugs which may be responsible and the treatment of nerve infiltration or compression. Where there is no reversible cause one of the membrane-stabilizing agents can be used. Quinine, 300 mg given at night, usually controls nocturnal cramps. Phenytoin or carbamazepine are useful in controlling daytime cramps. Corticosteroids can be of benefit in the neuropathic syndromes.

MUSCLE SPASM

Spasm secondary to bone disease. Painful bone metastases or pathological fractures are often associated with muscle spasm which serves to protect and splint the area. Treatment is directed at the underlying bone disease. Diazepam can be considered if the muscle spasm itself is causing significant pain.

Neuropathic spasm. Damage or disease in the brain or spinal cord can cause spasticity in the limbs which may be associated with painful muscle spasms. Treatment is of the causative pathology, if possible, and by physiotherapy. Troublesome muscle spasm can be treated with a skeletal muscle relaxant, although this may result in diminished mobility for the patient if there is reduction in muscle tone generally. Diazepam is given in the same dose as for anxiety; the main side effect is sedation. Baclofen acts at a spinal level but can also cause significant drowsiness. Dantrolene acts peripherally and is less likely to cause sedation.

MYOCLONUS

Myoclonus is involuntary twitching involving single muscles or muscle groups.

Cause (Table 7.3). Myoclonus can occur with any of the strong opioid drugs given in high doses, including morphine; it occurs more frequently with regular administration of meperidine. The myoclonus seen in dying patients may be a combination of organ failure and the effects of drugs.

Table 7.3 Causes of multifocal myoclonus

CNS disease	:	viral infection, paraneoplastic degenerative diseases
metabolic	:	hepatic or renal failure, hyponatremia, other
opioid drugs		
terminal phase		

Treatment. Myoclonus occurring with opioid therapy is treated by reducing the dose, if possible, or changing to an alternative drug. Reducing the opioid dose may also be considered in the terminal care situation if there is deteriorating renal function. Midazolam (2.5-10 mg SC, q2h until settled or 10-60 mg/24h SC infusion) is usually effective in controlling myoclonus.

HYPERTROPHIC PULMONARY OSTEOARTHROPATHY

Clinical features. Hypertrophic pulmonary osteoarthropathy (HPOA) is a paraneoplastic syndrome comprising clubbing of the fingers and toes, polyarthritis and periostitis. The joints most frequently involved are the wrists, ankles, knees and elbows; symptoms range from mild arthralgia to severe inflammatory arthritis. The patient complains of pain, tenderness and swelling over the affected bones and joints. X-ray examination shows periosteal reaction and isotopic bone scanning may be abnormal in these regions.

Treatment. Control of the underlying malignancy or treatment with NSAIDs usually produce significant improvement. HPOA also responds to bisphosphonate therapy.

BONE METASTASES

Clinical features. Bone metastases cause local pain. Initially, this may be intermittent, aggravated by movement and perhaps more noticeable at night. In weight bearing bones, pain is aggravated by standing and walking. There may be local tenderness to pressure or percussion. Bone metastases can be associated with a number of other clinical problems (Table 7.4).

Table 7.4 Bone metastases : clinical features

pain
impaired mobility and function
pathological fractures
hypercalcemia
spinal cord compression
nerve root compression
impaired bone marrow function

Assessment. The diagnosis of bone metastases is by x-ray and isotopic bone scanning. Bone scanning is more sensitive but less specific; abnormal scans may be seen with arthritis, infection, trauma and Paget's disease. Bone metastases can also be demonstrated on CT and MRI scanning, the latter being the method of choice for examination of the vertebral column.

Treatment

The aims of treatment are to relieve pain, prevent pathological fractures and to maintain or improve mobility and function (Table 7.5).

Table 7.5 Treatment options for bone metastases

analgesics	aspirin, NSAIDs, corticosteroids, opioids	*Treatment must be appropriate to the stage of the patient's disease and the prognosis*
systemic therapy	hormonal, chemotherapy (sensitive tumors)	
radiotherapy	local, hemibody, radioisotopes	
surgery	prophylaxis and fixation of fractures	
other	bisphosphonates	
physical	supports, mobility aids, physiotherapy	

Analgesics. Aspirin and NSAIDs are the analgesics of choice for the treatment of mild to moderate bone pain and are more effective than opioid drugs. When given for some other indication, corticosteroids may greatly reduce bone pain, probably by a similar mechanism. For more severe pain, opioid drugs are used in addition to the aspirin or NSAID.

Systemic therapy. Systemic therapy for sensitive tumors, if successful, will reduce bone pain.

Radiotherapy. Palliative radiotherapy for pain control will produce clinical improvement in about 80% of patients, whatever the histological type or tissue of origin of the tumor. Improvement occurs in 1-2 weeks and usually lasts for 3 to 4 months. Retreatment, if necessary, produces a similar response rate.

The optimal dose and fractionation for palliative radiotherapy should be the minimum effective dose given in the least number of treatment fractions. Prospective comparisons of standard therapy (e.g. 30 Gy in 10-15 fractions) with lower doses (e.g. 8 Gy in 1-2 fractions) have shown no differences in the proportion of patients achieving pain control or the duration of response. Vertebral metastases associated with, or threatening, spinal cord compression are better treated with longer courses of therapy in order to avoid the acute edema associated with larger fractions and because the goal of treatment may be tumor shrinkage as well as pain control.

Hemibody irradiation (HBI). Hemibody irradiation should be considered for patients with widespread painful metastases. A single dose is given to the upper, lower or mid-part of the body; the maximum tolerable dose to the lower half of the body is 8 Gy, 6 Gy for the upper half. If necessary, the other half can be treated 4-8 weeks later, after recovery of myelosuppression. HBI does not prevent further local radiotherapy being given to local painful areas. HBI is effective in controlling pain in 80-85% of patients treated and the response does not depend on the histological type or tissue of origin of the tumor. The majority of patients respond within 48 hours and the median duration of response is 4 months.

The toxicity of HBI is considerable and includes nausea, vomiting and diarrhea, myelosuppression, mucositis, pneumonitis and alopecia.   HBI is therefore not appropriate for patients with significantly reduced blood counts, those in generally poor physical condition or with a life expectancy of less than 2 months.

Radiopharmaceuticals. Strontium (^{89}Sr) is used to treat widespread metastases. It is best for tumors which have markedly increased osteoblastic activity, with sclerotic changes on x-ray, as is seen with prostate and some breast cancers. About 80% of patients treated with strontium will respond, improvement occurring after 10 to 20 days and lasting 4 to 6 months. Strontium also delays the onset of bone pain in new areas for a period of about four months although it has no effect on survival.

Strontium therapy is well tolerated.   The only significant side effect is myelosuppression which is usually mild and not clinically significant. However, patients with severely compromised bone marrow function for other reasons should not be treated with strontium. The disadvantage of strontium is its considerable cost.

Surgery. Surgery is employed for the prevention and treatment of pathological fractures. Prophylactic surgery is most frequently used for metastatic disease involving the neck or shaft of the femur. Radiographic assessment alone cannot adequately identify all lesions at high risk of fracture, but some general guidelines are listed in Table 7.6. Surgical fixation provides prompt pain relief and allows early mobilization and rehabilitation.

Table 7.6 Bone metastases : some indications for prophylactic surgery

medullary lesion :	>50% diameter of the bone
cortical lesion :	destruction of >50% of cortical width
	axial length > diameter of bone
	> 2-3 cm
any lesion causing pain unrelieved by radiotherapy	

Bisphosphonates. The bisphosphonate compounds are pyrophosphate analogues which inhibit bone resorption and are useful in the treatment of hypercalcemia. Pamidronate will improve pain control in about 60% of patients with bone metastases and also reduce the incidence of hypercalcemia, pathological fractures and the development of new areas of bone pain. The usual dose is pamidronate 60-90 mg in 500 ml of saline or dextrose, infused over 1-2 hours, each 4 weeks. The dose should be reduced or administered more slowly in patients with significant renal impairment. A few patients may suffer mild nausea or develop a low grade fever. A number of more potent bisphosphonates are likely to be available in the future.

Terminal care. The treatment of bone metastases in the last days or week of life should be directed solely at patient comfort. Because of the uncertainty of estimating life expectancy, palliative radiotherapy needs to be considered if the pain is difficult to control and may be effective within days. Surgical procedures are usually not indicated. Splinting and skin traction may be of benefit. Adequate analgesia needs to be prescribed, including extra doses to be given before moving or turning the patient.

Further Reading – see page 111

8 Dermatological

cutaneous manifestations of cancer   fungating tumors
pruritus   pressure sores
herpes zoster   radiotherapy reactions

CUTANEOUS MANIFESTATIONS OF CANCER

Recognition of these clinical syndromes allows the patient to be reassured and, in some cases, symptomatic treatment applied.

Xerosis. Dry, fine scaling of the skin is common in patients with advanced cancer. Treatment is symptomatic with topical moisturising medication.

Acquired ichthyosis. The entire skin is dry with rhomboidal scales and hyperkeratotic palms and soles. Treatment is with emollients to keep the skin as moist as possible; if scaling is severe, a keratolytic such as 2% salicylic acid can be added to the emollient.

Acanthosis nigricans. The development of velvety brown hyperkeratotic plaques in the flexures of the axillae, groins and neck has a strong association with internal malignancy. It can also involve the periareolar and periumbilical area.

Hypertrichosis lanuginosa. This is characterized by the development of fine, silky lanugo-like hair ('malignant down'), first affecting the face and later the entire body surface.

Dermatomyositis. Dermatomyositis is the association of progressive proximal muscle weakness with a purplish pink photosensitive erythema involving the exposed parts of the face, neck and backs of the hands which occurs in association with internal malignancy. It sometimes improves with treatment of the underlying tumor and can also respond to systemic corticosteroids or immunosuppression.

Hyperpigmentation. Diffuse hyperpigmentation may occur in Cushing's syndrome and with ectopic ACTH production by tumors. A few patients with disseminated melanoma develop a generalized slate-grey discoloration.

Erythema ab igne. Areas of reticulated (lace-net-like) brown discoloration are seen commonly in patients with advanced cancer, due to the frequent self-application of hot water bottles or heating pads to relieve pain.

PRURITUS

Cause (Table 8.1).

Treatment

Therapy is symptomatic and, if possible, by treatment of the underlying cause.

Treatment of specific causes. Extrahepatic obstruction can be treated by stent insertion, bypass surgery or radiotherapy; intrahepatic obstruction due to tumor may improve with corticosteroids. Cholestyramine (4g PO, 6-hourly) can reduce pruritus in patients with cholestasis but is unpalatable. Therapy with an androgenic steroid may relieve pruritus associated with cholestasis, often within a few days. A variety of other

Table 8.1 Causes of generalized pruritus

cholestasis	skin disease
malignant obstruction	drug reactions
drugs	radiotherapy reactions
hepatitis	ichthyosis
renal failure	infections : scabies, candida
malignancy	atopic dermatitis
polycythemia vera	urticaria
other myeloproliferative disorders	endocrine disorders
Hodgkin's disease	thyroid disease
other lymphomas	diabetes
intraspinal morphine	
iron deficiency	

agents are reported to be effective including the $5HT_3$ receptor antagonist, ondansetron. Drugs suspected of causing cholestasis should be stopped. Pruritus associated with uremia responds to dialysis or treatment with erythropoietin. Primary skin disorders are treated appropriately. Pruritus associated with intraspinal morphine responds poorly to antihistamines; treatment with naloxone or subhypnotic doses of propofol are reported to be effective.

Topical therapy. A cool or air conditioned environment will reduce sweating and lessen itch. Hot baths and substances which cause vasodilatation (alcohol, hot drinks) are avoided. Calamine lotion, or menthol and camphor creams act by cooling the skin. Topical anesthetic agents and topical corticosteroid applications are helpful for some patients.

Antihistamines. Antihistamines are most effective for pruritus due to allergy and are often much less effective in treating pruritus due to other causes. The use of antihistamines is limited by sedation There is considerable individual variation with regard to the effects and side effects of the various antihistamines and it is customary to trial other agents if the drug chosen first is ineffective (Table 8.2). A trial of corticosteroids (prednisolone 25-50 mg/d) can be considered in patients with severe or intractable pruritus.

Table 8.2 Examples of antihistamine drugs used for pruritus

antihistamine	
diphenhydramine	25-50 mg q6h
chlorpheniramine	4 mg q6h
plus phenothiazine action	
trimeprazine	10 mg q8h
promethazine	20-50 mg q12h
chlorpromazine	25-50 mg q6h
plus anxiolytic action	
hydroxyzine	10-25 mg q8-12h
plus antiserotonin action	
cyproheptadine	4 mg q8-12h

HERPES ZOSTER

Herpes zoster or shingles is caused by the varicella zoster virus (VZV).

Clinical features. Herpes zoster presents as a unilateral vesicular rash in a dermatomal distribution. It occurs most commonly in the thoracic region and on the face and neck. Acute herpes zoster is associated with pain which can precede the appearance of the rash by one or two days. The rash normally dries and subsides spontaneously in two to four weeks. Cutaneous dissemination causes a rash similar to varicella or chickenpox while visceral dissemination can manifest as encephalitis, transverse myelitis, hepatitis or pneumonitis.

Treatment

Antiviral therapy. Antiviral therapy (Table 8.3) started within 48 hours of the appearance of the rash will reduce acute pain, improve the rate of healing and reduce the risk of dissemination; whether it reduces the incidence of postherpetic neuralgia is unresolved. Herpes zoster involving the eye requires therapy with topical aciclovir and corticosteroids and should be assessed by an ophthalmologist.

Table 8.3 Herpes zoster : antiviral therapy*

---
standard therapy
    aciclovir 800 mg PO, 5 times daily for 7 days
    famciclovir 250 mg PO, 3 times daily for 7 days
intensive therapy (multiple dermatomes, signs suggestive of dissemination)
    aciclovir 10 mg/kg IV q8h for 7 days

---

    * dose reductions required if there is renal impairment

Topical therapy. Topical treatment of the rash is symptomatic and includes saline-soaked gauze pads or Burow's solution (aluminum acetate) for early, weeping lesions and calamine lotion for pruritic, healing lesions. Secondary infection should be treated appropriately.

Postherpetic neuralgia. A small proportion of patients develop persisting pain in the affected dermatome which responds poorly to standard non-opioid and opioid analgesics. Treatment with an antidepressant or anticonvulsant is more likely to be effective. Resistant neuralgia sometimes responds to TENS, acupuncture or epidural injection of corticosteroid. The topical application of 0.025% capsaicin cream is of benefit in some patients.

FUNGATING TUMORS

Clinical features. Fungation of cancer through the skin causes disfigurement and pain and is frequently associated with infection and odor.

Treatment

Radiotherapy. Palliative radiotherapy is considered for all fungating lesions and can produce significant tumor shrinkage and relief of symptoms.

Systemic therapy. Hormonal treatment or chemotherapy may be of benefit for patients with sensitive tumors.

Miltefosine. Miltefosine is a novel anticancer agent which probably interacts with the cancer cell membrane rather than DNA. Topical application leads to regression of skin lesions in a proportion of women with breast cancer; it may also have activity against cutaneous lymphoma and skin metastases from melanoma. It is most effective for small superficial lesions. Miltefosine is applied daily for the first week, then twice daily, for eight weeks. Side effects are generally mild and include pruritus and erythema; local discomfort or burning occur more frequently if the lesions are ulcerated.

Topical therapy. Fungating tumors require frequent and regular dressings, the aim being to keep the area clean, dry and free of infection. If the surface is clean, it is simply washed with normal saline. Dead and sloughing tissue is removed with a dilute solution of hydrogen peroxide and saline. Bleeding is less likely if alginate dressings are used and can be controlled by applying gauze soaked in epinephrine 1:1000. The lesion is dressed with a melonin or other nonadherent dressing which needs to be sufficiently absorbent to soak up any exudate. The dressing is held in place with tubular elastic netting.

Odor control. The application of metronidazole gel will control anaerobic infection and reduce odor. If unsuccessful, systemic metronidazole (400 mg PO, 8-hourly) is frequently of benefit; an alternative is clindamycin (150 mg PO, 6-hourly). Charcoal pads placed under the netting holding the dressing will further reduce odor.

PRESSURE SORES

Cause. Pressure sores are caused by tissue ischemia due to pressure, usually over bony prominences. A considerable number of other factors predispose to the development of pressure sores (Table 8.4).

Table 8.4 Factors predisposing to pressure sores

tissue damage
    pressure
    friction, shearing forces : improper skin care
    urine, feces, excess moisture
    infection
    direct tissue injury : burns, injections, crumpled bed clothes
    restlessness
tissue fragility/poor repair
    weight loss, emaciation
    old age
    malnourishment : protein, vitamin C, zinc
    anemia, vascular insufficiency, edema
    corticosteroids
    chemotherapy, radiotherapy
immobility
    weakness, paralysis, general debility
    sedation or impaired consciousness
    positioning for treatment of other pressure areas
diminished response to pain or irritation
    hypoesthesia, anesthesia
    analgesics
    sedation or impaired consciousness

Clinical features. A classification based on the visible depth of tissue damage provides a logical basis for treatment (Table 8.5).

Table 8.5 Pressure sores

Level 1	skin intact
	blanching or non-blanching erythema
	soft tissue swelling and induration
Level 2	skin broken
	shallow ulceration or skin loss involving epidermis or dermis
	vesicles, blebs
Level 3	ulceration involving subcutaneous fatty tissue
	necrotic tissue, eschar formation common
Level 4	ulceration involving fascia, muscle or bone
	necrotic tissue, eschar formation common

Treatment

While theoretically preventable, the development of pressure sores in some terminally ill patients is unavoidable and does not necessarily indicate inadequate nursing. The combination of immobility, emaciation, poor nutrition and incontinence can make the prevention of pressure sores almost impossible. For the same reasons, all but superficial pressure ulcers may be difficult to heal in the terminally ill.

Preventive. The treatment of pressure sores is, wherever possible, preventive. Patients at risk of developing pressure sores should be identified and a range of preventive measures initiated (Table 8.6).

Table 8.6 Prevention of pressure sores

identify patients at risk	
general hygiene	keep skin clean and dry
avoid trauma	pat or blow skin dry, avoid rubbing
	avoid vigorous massage
	lift patients, avoid dragging
	avoid wet clothes, bedding
	avoid contamination with urine, feces
	avoid rough garments, bedding
	avoid excess heat (lamps)
	avoid crumpled bedclothes
	avoid harsh soaps, alcohol rubs
avoid friction	sheepskin mats and boots to reduce friction
relief of pressure	frequent turning, repositioning
	correct positioning
	special mattresses
general	optimize nutrition
	avoid corticosteroids, sedation, excess analgesics

Active treatment. The treatment of pressure sores needs to be appropriate to the stage of the patient's disease. For patients with shorter life expectancy or extensive ulceration, energetic therapy stands little, if any, chance of healing the lesion. A balance must be found between the anticipated morbidity from the lesion and the inconvenience of treatment (Table 8.7).

Terminal care. The treatment of pressure sores in terminally ill patients is symptomatic. Frequent turning and other measures designed to allow healing are irrelevant, especially if movement causes pain.

Table 8.7 Treatment of pressure sores

relieve pressure	
local hygiene	saline
	topical antiseptics (short term only)
debridement	enzymatic e.g. collagenase, Elase
	hydrophilic substances : dextranomer (Debrisan)
	surgical
promote healing	superficial : semipermeable membrane
	deeper : impermeable hydrocolloid dressing
systemic antibiotics	for cellulitis, osteomyelitis
analgesics	as required for pain
reduce odor	topical metronidazole gel, charcoal dressings

RADIOTHERAPY SKIN REACTIONS

Radiotherapy skin reactions are more likely with higher doses, doses delivered more quickly and in normally moist areas such as the perineum, axilla or inframammary fold.

Acute. In the acute stage there will be erythema and edema associated with pruritus. This is followed by desquamation, alopecia and loss of sweating (anhidrosis). These changes usually resolve spontaneously over several months. During the acute phase, care should be taken to avoid any mechanical, chemical or thermal injury to the affected skin (Table 8.8).

Table 8.8 Management of acute radiation skin reactions

general	loose, soft, non-synthetic clothing
	wash gently in lukewarm water, dry gently
	avoid perfumes, soaps, powders, lotions or deodorants which may contain irritating chemicals
	protection from sun with sunscreens
dry reaction	baby oil, lanolin ointment or non-irritating moisturizing cream
	hydrocortisone 1% cream if severe
moist reaction	keep clean and dry, treat secondary infection
	bathe with aluminum acetate (Burow's solution)
	povidone-iodine or silver sulfadiazine for infected areas

Chronic. In the chronic phase, the skin is thin and atrophic and there may be hypo- or hyper-pigmentation and cutaneous telangiectasia. In more severe cases there may be necrosis and ulceration.

Radiation recall phenomenon. Acute skin reactions may occur in previously irradiated areas following the administration of chemotherapy drugs. The exact explanation is unknown. Treatment is as for acute skin reactions.

Further Reading - see page 111

9   Neurological

> **cerebral metastases**
> **recurrent cerebral tumors**
> **spinal cord compression**
> **meningeal tumor infiltration**
> **seizures**
> **acute confusion or delirium**
>
> **terminal restlessness**
> **dementia**
> **insomnia**
> **paraneoplastic syndromes**
> **eye problems**

CEREBRAL METASTASES

Clinical features. Symptoms and signs of cerebral metastases are due to focal disruption of neurological function, mechanical pressure and displacement of tissue, and raised intracranial pressure (Table 9.1). The natural history of cerebral metastases is progressive neurological deterioration with a median life expectancy of 1 to 2 months. The neurological disabilities, particularly of cognitive and motor function, can have a profound effect on the quality of life.

Assessment. The diagnosis is made on CT or MRI scanning.

Table 9.1 Clinical features of cerebral metastases

Symptoms	Signs
headache	cognitive impairment
weakness : focal or hemiparetic	hemiparesis
mental state changes	sensory loss : focal or unilateral
behavioral, personality changes	loss of co-ordination, ataxia
seizures	papilledema
loss of co-ordination, ataxia	aphasia
aphasia	

Treatment

The goal of treatment is to restore and maintain neurological function or at least to minimize deterioration. The treatment options are listed in Table 9.2.

Corticosteroids. Dexamethasone 16-24 mg/day will produce clinical improvement in 60-80% of patients with cerebral metastases. The effect is seen usually within the first 24 hours, with 2 to 3 days taken for maximal effect. Corticosteroids are more effective against generalized neurological features (e.g. headaches, confusion) than against focal neurological dysfunction (e.g. hemiparesis). Patients who do not respond to standard doses may benefit from a higher dose, although the chances of a clinically meaningful response are small. If there is no improvement after 7 days, the dose should

Table 9.2 Treatment for cerebral metastases

specific therapy	symptomatic care	
corticosteroids	anticonvulsants	*Treatment must be*
radiotherapy	physical therapy	*appropriate to the stage*
surgery	psychological therapy	*of the patient's disease*
systemic therapy (sensitive tumors)		*and the prognosis*

be reduced as much as possible. Patients responding to corticosteroid therapy should also have the dose reduced to the lowest effective dose although those proceeding with radiotherapy may have it continued to lessen the side effects of irradiation.

Radiotherapy. Patients with cerebral metastases are treated with radiotherapy, provided the state of their systemic disease and the degree of neurological dysfunction make such therapy appropriate. Patients who have responded well to corticosteroids are more likely to benefit from radiotherapy, as the initial response indicates that more of the clinical features were due to reversible edema and raised intracranial pressure than to irreversible destruction of brain tissue. Shorter courses of treatment are employed for cerebral metastases than for primary brain tumors. The response rate is equivalent and the shorter courses are less troublesome for the patient. Whole brain or cranial irradiation is given because of the high incidence of multiple metastases. About two thirds of patients with cerebral metastases selected to receive radiotherapy will show clinical improvement. The median survival of patients treated in this manner is 3 to 6 months.

Surgery. Surgical resection of metastatic disease is of benefit to a small number of carefully selected patients. Eligibility requires a surgically accessible solitary metastasis and a good performance status in a patient with no or controllable disease at other sites. Surgery is usually followed by radiotherapy and this combined treatment has been shown to prolong survival and reduce the risk of neurological relapse. Surgery may also be required for the relief of obstructive hydrocephalus by the insertion of a ventriculo-atrial shunt.

Systemic therapy. Hormonal therapy for hormone-sensitive tumors may be effective in controlling cerebral disease. Chemotherapy for cerebral metastases has generally disappointing results as the agents do not freely cross the blood brain barrier.

Anticonvulsants. Anticonvulsant therapy is given to any patient who has had a seizure. The prophylactic use of anticonvulsants for all patients with cerebral metastases is not warranted as only about 20% will suffer a seizure.

Physical therapy. Patients with motor or sensory deficits or problems of co-ordination require appropriate physiotherapy and rehabilitation. The patient and family need help adjusting to neurological deficits and the use of physical aids and modifications to the patient's immediate environment at home are important.

Psychological therapy. Patients with cerebral metastases may have labile mood, personality alteration, depression and anxiety as well as impairment of cognitive function. Treatment includes the appropriate use of anxiolytics, antidepressants, tranquillizers and hypnotics as well as supportive counselling for both the patient and the family.

Treatment of herniation. Emergency measures to control raised intracranial pressure and prevent cerebral herniation are only appropriate if it is considered that active therapy for the underlying cerebral metastatic disease will result in significant clinical benefit. Measures include elevation of the patient's head, high dose dexamethasone (24 mg IV), mannitol (25-100 g IV) and mechanical hyperventilation to reduce cerebral blood flow by reducing the pCO_2.

Terminal care. Patients whose life expectancy is very short because of the effects of disease at other sites are appropriately treated with analgesics and antiemetics. Corticosteroids can be considered if seizures or headache are difficult to control. Radiotherapy is not indicated for terminally ill patients. Patients lapsing into coma can have their corticosteroids discontinued unless seizures are difficult to control.

RECURRENT CEREBRAL TUMORS

Clinical features. Patients with recurrent primary brain tumors present similar clinical features to those with cerebral metastases but are more likely to have significant physical disability, cognitive impairment and psychological disturbance, due to the combined effects of recurrent tumor and previous therapy. They are frequently severely Cushingoid from chronic corticosteroid administration.

Treatment. Treatment is symptomatic and the options are few. Surgery is rarely indicated unless obstructive hydrocephalus develops. Increasing the dose of corticosteroid is often of limited clinical benefit. Further radiotherapy is usually not feasible. Treatment is with analgesics and antiemetics, psychological counselling and the appropriate use of psychotropic medications, physiotherapy and physical supports, delivered as part of a co-ordinated overall plan of supportive care for the patient and the family.

SPINAL CORD COMPRESSION

Cause. Spinal cord compression is usually caused by extradural extension of tumor from an involved vertebra. Rarely, compression occurs from epidural or spinal cord metastases occurring without bone involvement. Rapid onset or progression of spinal cord signs over a period of several hours, with complete loss of neurological function, is usually due to cord infarction and is irreversible.

Clinical features. Pain is the initial symptom in more than 90% of patients and can precede the development of neurological dysfunction by days or months. Vertebral involvement causes central back pain, aggravated by movement or coughing and usually associated with local tenderness. Nerve root irritation produces unilateral or bilateral radicular pain. Plain x-rays show evidence of vertebral involvement in most patients.

Spinal cord compression produces progressive weakness and sensory loss, as well as constipation and urinary retention. Examination shows sensory loss and motor weakness with reduced muscle tone. Reflexes are reduced or absent. Anal tone is reduced or absent and the bladder may be distended.

Assessment. MRI scanning is non-invasive and provides the most information. The site and extent of the lesion causing compression can be determined and, as the whole spine is imaged, other deposits causing or potentially causing extradural compression can be identified. If MRI scanning is inconclusive or unavailable, myelography with CT scanning should be performed. Raised intracranial pressure (due to cerebral metastases) needs to be excluded by clinical examination and CT scanning before the lumbar puncture for myelography is performed. If the myelogram shows only a partial subarachnoid block, the upper limit of the lesion causing compression can be defined and other lesions excluded; if there is a complete block, a cervical or cisternal myelogram has to be considered to define the upper limit of the lesion and to exclude multiple lesions. The cerebrospinal fluid is examined for malignant cells.

Treatment

The primary aim of treatment is to maximize the recovery of neurological function. Secondary to this are the goals of local tumor control, pain control and spinal stability. An approach to the management of spinal cord compression is shown in Figure 9.1.

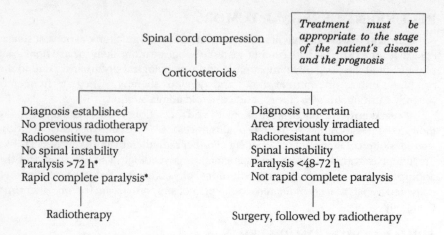

Figure 9.1 of spinal cord compression content:

Spinal cord compression

| Treatment must be appropriate to the stage of the patient's disease and the prognosis |

Corticosteroids

Diagnosis established
No previous radiotherapy
Radiosensitive tumor
No spinal instability
Paralysis >72 h*
Rapid complete paralysis*

Radiotherapy

Diagnosis uncertain
Area previously irradiated
Radioresistant tumor
Spinal instability
Paralysis <48-72 h
Not rapid complete paralysis

Surgery, followed by radiotherapy

*radiotherapy indicated for local pain or tumor control; neurological recovery most unlikely

Figure 9.1   Management of spinal cord compression

Urgency. Spinal cord compression is considered an emergency because the single most important determinant of neurological outcome is the degree of neurological impairment at the time of starting therapy. About 80% of ambulatory patients, but only 45% of non-ambulatory ones, will be able to walk after treatment and less than 10% of paraplegic patients will become ambulatory.

Corticosteroids. Dexamethasone (12-24 mg IV initially, followed by 24 mg/d) is given as soon as a diagnosis of spinal cord compression is made or suspected.

Radiotherapy. Radiotherapy is the standard treatment for malignant cord compression. Neurological deterioration during radiotherapy is an indication for surgery. The neurological results of treatment with dexamethasone plus radiotherapy are equivalent to dexamethasone and laminectomy plus radiotherapy.

Surgery. Patients showing rapid neurological deterioration are treated by urgent posterior laminectomy, although tumor removal is incomplete and it can contribute to spinal instability. Anterior decompression laminectomy with spinal stabilization can be considered for selected patients with a solitary lesion, good performance status, good neurological status before treatment and controllable disease at other sites. It is reported to provide better decompression, spinal stability and local pain control. It is customary to follow surgical decompression with radiotherapy and rapid mobilization is encouraged.

Surgery is not indicated for patients with established paraplegia (>72 hours), those in whom complete paralysis developed rapidly over a few hours due to cord infarction, or those who are severely debilitated or have restricted mobility.

Paraplegia. Patients with permanent paralysis require a program of rehabilitation and supportive care. This includes bowel, bladder and skin care as well as physiotherapy, the use of aids and physical alterations to the home environment.

Terminal care. The development of spinal cord compression during the last days or week of life should be treated with analgesia and supportive care; dexamethasone may be of symptomatic benefit.

MENINGEAL TUMOR INFILTRATION

Clinical features. Meningeal tumor infiltration characteristically produces neurological dysfunction at multiple levels. Cerebral features include headache, nausea and vomiting, lethargy, confusion and mental state changes. Cranial nerve lesions are common and frequently multiple. Spinal features include back pain, motor weakness and unsteadiness, radicular pain, numbness and autonomic dysfunction with loss of bowel and bladder function; the spinal features may mimic extradural spinal cord compression. The natural history of meningeal tumor infiltration is one of progressive neurological deterioration.

Assessment. CT or MRI scanning may be normal or show meningeal thickening or nodularity; hydrocephalus without evidence of a mass lesion is another common finding. Examination of cerebrospinal fluid will show malignant cells in most patients.

Treatment

General. Corticosteroids can improve symptoms and there may be transient improvement in neurological function. Obstructive hydrocephalus can be relieved by the insertion of a shunt.

Radiotherapy. Local radiotherapy can be given to areas of symptomatic or bulky disease and may improve neurological function.

Chemotherapy. Chemotherapy for meningeal infiltration needs to be given intrathecally by lumbar puncture or via an Ommaya reservoir, as systemic chemotherapy is usually ineffective. Intrathecal chemotherapy is frequently effective against hematological malignancies but will produce improvement in only one third of patients with relatively chemosensitive solid tumors such as small cell lung or breast cancer; the response rate for other solid tumors is even lower.

Hormone therapy. Systemic hormonal therapy may be effective in controlling meningeal infiltration by sensitive tumors.

Terminal care. Meningeal infiltration in the terminally ill is treated symptomatically with analgesics, antiemetics and supportive care. Dexamethasone may aid the palliation of symptoms.

SEIZURES

Cause (Table 9.3). Seizures occur in 20% of patients with cerebral metastases.

Table 9.3 Causes of seizures

tumor	primary, metastatic, meningeal infiltration
	hemorrhage, obstructive hydrocephalus
infection	bacterial, fungal, parasitic, viral
metabolic	hepatic encephalopathy, uremia, hypoglycemia, hyponatremia
drug toxicity	meperidine, tricyclic antidepressants, phenothiazines, local anesthetics
drug withdrawal	benzodiazepines, barbiturates, alcohol

Clinical features. The clinical features of generalized seizures in patients with cancer are the same as seen in patients with epilepsy. The tonic-clonic phase can be preceded by focal (Jacksonian) features which may be progressive, starting with twitching in the hand, foot or face, progressing centrally and culminating in a typical tonic-clonic seizure. Transient motor weakness may follow a seizure (Todd's paresis).

Assessment. For patients with documented cerebral metastases, investigations may be considered unnecessary. In the absence of known CNS disease, a brain scan and other appropriate investigations should be performed.

Treatment

Drug therapy. Treatment with a benzodiazepine is given following a generalized seizure to reduce the risk of a second convulsion (Table 9.4). However, the anticonvulsant action is short lived and other therapy should be instituted promptly. Phenytoin is the most frequently used anticonvulsant and the dose should be adjusted according to blood levels. Alternatively, if therapy is likely to be short term, blood levels need only be checked if the patient has more seizures or there are signs of toxicity. Elderly and debilitated patients and those with impaired liver function are at increased risk of toxicity. Patients requiring continuing anticonvulsant therapy who are unable to take oral medication because of dysphagia, vomiting or unconsciousness may be treated with midazolam by subcutaneous infusion or rectal diazepam.

Table 9.4 Management of seizures

Immediate therapy to reduce the risk of a second seizure
    diazepam 10 mg IV or PR (rectal enema) *or*
    midazolam 10 mg IV or SC
Standard anticonvulsant therapy with phenytoin
    loading dose : 1000 mg (or 15-20 mg/kg) PO in divided doses over 24h
    maintenance : 300-400 mg (or 5-6 mg/kg)/d PO, adjusted according to blood levels
    side effects : sedation, cognitive impairment, ataxia, dysarthria, nystagmus
    drug interactions : common
    alternatives : carbamazepine, clonazepam
Status epilepticus
    diazepam 10-20 mg IV (at <5mg/min), *followed by*
    phenytoin 15-20 mg/kg IV (at <50 mg/min)
Treatment for patients unable to take oral medications
    diazepam 10 mg PR q12h *or*
    midazolam 10-30 mg/24h SC infusion and titrate

Counselling. Patients suffering seizures require counselling as for any patient with epilepsy. A seizure may be the first sign of progressive or metastatic disease and cause considerable distress for the patient and family. Patients with cerebral metastases who have suffered a seizure are instructed not to drive a motor vehicle, both for reasons of safety and because most insurance policies are invalid should an accident occur.

Status epilepticus. Patients who do not recover consciousness between seizures are treated as a medical emergency. Treatment is with intravenous diazepam or clonazepam followed by phenytoin (Table 9.4).

Terminal care. At some stage during the terminal phase, patients will no longer be able to take oral anticonvulsant medication. For patients who have had no recent seizures, the medication should be stopped. Patients requiring continued therapy are treated with midazolam by subcutaneous infusion or rectal diazepam.

ACUTE CONFUSION OR DELIRIUM

Cause (Table 9.5). In many cases confusion is due to more than one cause. Drug toxicity is a frequent and reversible cause of confusion and is more likely in elderly or frail patients. In addition, there are a number of contributing factors which may precipitate or aggravate an acute confusional state or delirium (Table 9.6).

Table 9.5 Causes of acute confusion or delirium

intracranial pathology
    tumor, hemorrhage, obstructive hydrocephalus, infection, encephalopathy (radiation, chemotherapy), post seizure, paraneoplastic syndromes
metabolic
    respiratory failure (hypoxia, hypercapnia), hepatic failure, renal failure, electrolyte disorder (hyponatremia, hypercalcemia, acidosis, alkalosis), endocrine (hypoglycemia, hyperglycemia, adrenal and thyroid dysfunction)
infection, fever
drugs
    alcohol, anticholinergics, anticonvulsants, antidepressants, antiemetics, antihistamines, antiparkinsonian agents, antipsychotics (chlorpromazine, haloperidol), anxiolytics and hypnotics (barbiturates, benzodiazepines), corticosteroids, NSAIDs, opioid analgesics, stimulants (amphetamine, methylphenidate, cocaine) and, less frequently, many other drugs
drug withdrawal
    alcohol, barbiturate, benzodiazepine, nicotine, opioids
circulatory
    dehydration, hypovolemia, hyperviscosity, cerebrovascular disease, anemia

Table 9.6 Acute confusion or delirium : contributing factors

anxiety	pre-existing cerebral disease, dementia
depression	general debility
pain, discomfort	sleep deprivation
altered environment	

Clinical features. Acute confusion or delirium may be acute or subacute, developing over hours or days. The clinical features are listed in Table 9.7. The first signs include restlessness with periods of disorientation and there may be impaired short term memory. Acute confusional states characteristically fluctuate and there may be lucid intervals. The condition invariably becomes worse in the evening and at night. The cardinal sign is that there has been a change in the mental or psychological state from a short time previously.

Table 9.7 Acute confusional state or delirium : clinical features

altered conscious state	drowsy, semiconscious, reduced awareness
	may be hyperactive
attention deficit	poor concentration
altered mood (affect)	terrified, euphoric, paranoid
impaired short term memory	
impaired thinking	
impaired judgement	
altered perception	misperceptions, misinterpretations, illusions
	delusions (usually paranoid), hallucinations
disorientation	time, place, other persons
speech	rambling, incoherent
disturbed sleep pattern	drowsy by day, insomnia at night
abnormal behavior	hyperactive - often aimless, repetitive
	hypoactive - lethargic, catatonic
abnormal psychomotor activity	hyperactive - restless, irritable, aggressive, noisy
	hypoactive - withdrawn, stupor
clinical course	acute or subacute onset, fluctuating course
	nocturnal exacerbation

Assessment (Table 9.8). Assessment includes general physical, neurological and mental state examinations. Mental state examination includes assessment of the patient's mood and affect, orientation, thought content, short term memory and other intellectual functions. Other investigations can be considered, depending on the results of clinical assessment and the severity of the symptoms.

Table 9.8 Assessment of acute confusion or delirium

knowledge of
    previous mental state
    previous psychiatric disorder
    previous alcohol or drug abuse

> *Investigation must be appropriate to the stage of the patient's disease and the prognosis*

examination
    physical, neurological, mental
assess recent and current drug administration
laboratory tests
    electrolytes and renal function, liver function tests, serum calcium, blood sugar, arterial
        blood gases and pH, coagulation profile and platelet count, bacteriological cultures
CT or MRI scan
CSF examination

Treatment

Treatment of the cause. The underlying cause (Table 9.5) should be sought and treated, where possible and appropriate. Medications causing acute confusion should be reduced or stopped, provided good symptom and pain control are maintained. If confusion is caused by alcohol or drug withdrawal a case can be made, especially in the terminally ill, for allowing the patient to continue to take the offending agent; nicotine withdrawal can be treated with nicotine skin patches.

General measures. The provision of an appropriate physical environment and good nursing care are the cornerstone of management of most patients with mild confusion. The patient's room needs to be quiet and well lit; a night light should be available. Repeated calm reassurance and explanation, minimizing the number of different staff having contact with the patient, the presence of a family member or trusted friend, avoidance of disruptive disturbances and the development of a regular daily routine may all lessen, or at least not aggravate, a patient's confusion. A confused patient should not be moved from familiar surroundings unless absolutely necessary. Physical restraints are avoided if possible. Restless patients can be allowed to ambulate if accompanied; habitual smokers should be allowed to smoke with supervision. Anxiety and depression, if present, are treated appropriately, provided that any drug measures used do not complicate the confusional state.

Drug therapy. Haloperidol is used for treatment of delirium in medically ill patients. The dose required varies with the patient's physical state and the severity of their symptoms. Most patients will improve on haloperidol 1-5 mg, 8-hourly, given orally or subcutaneously. Severely agitated, aggressive or psychotic patients may require 5-10 mg by injection, repeated hourly and titrated against effect. Haloperidol therapy can be continued either orally or by subcutaneous infusion. If sedation is necessary to lessen agitation, midazolam 5-10 mg subcutaneously, 2-hourly, can be given with haloperidol and therapy continued by continuous subcutaneous infusion. Chlorpromazine, which is more sedating than haloperidol, is an alternative.

TERMINAL RESTLESSNESS

Clinical features. Terminal restlessness is a particular variant of acute confusion or delirium which occurs in some patients during their last few days of life. The clinical features are listed in Table 9.9. Family members may be upset by terminal restlessness, particularly if there is moaning, grunting or other distressed vocalizing.

Table 9.9 Terminal restlessness

agitation	muscle twitching
impaired conscious state	multifocal myoclonus
distressed vocalizing	seizures

Assessment. Restlessness due to anxiety or fear, unrelieved pain, urinary retention or fecal impaction and drug, alcohol or nicotine withdrawal should be excluded. The use of opioid analgesics needs to be reviewed, as they may cause or aggravate myoclonus in terminally ill patients with deteriorating renal function.

Treatment

Treatment is by sedation, usually with a benzodiazepine (Table 9.10). Midazolam has the advantage that it can be given by continuous subcutaneous infusion but there is considerable variation in the effective dose which can lead to significant delays in achieving control for patients requiring higher doses. Sublingual lorazepam may be effective but is short acting. Another alternative which can be helpful in the home care situation is to give rectal temazepam by making a needle hole through the oral capsule and inserting it as a suppository. Haloperidol should be used if benzodiazepine therapy is unsuccessful.

Table 9.10 Treatment of terminal restlessness

benzodiazepines
diazepam	10-20 mg PR, q4-6h and titrate
midazolam	2.5-10 mg SC, q2h or 60 mg/24h SC infusion and titrate
lorazepam	1-2.5 mg SL, q2-4h and titrate
temazepam	10-20 mg PR, q6-8h and titrate

for benzodiazepine failure
haloperidol	5-30 mg/24h SC infusion and titrate

DEMENTIA

Cause (Table 9.11). Dementia in patients with cancer is unrelated to the cancer or treatment in 85% of cases.

Clinical features (Table 9.12). Patients with dementia are more prone to develop an acute confusional state if subject to any of the causes or contributing factors shown in Tables 9.5 and 9.6.

Table 9.11 Causes of dementia

unrelated to cancer or treatment
  Alzheimer's disease
  alcoholic dementia
  cerebrovascular disease
  other : hydrocephalus, thyroid dysfunction, vitamin deficiency, infection
related to cancer or treatment
  malignant infiltration, obstructive hydrocephalus
  radiotherapy
  chemotherapy
  infection
  paraneoplastic syndromes

Table 9.12 Dementia : clinical features

onset	insidious
course	little fluctuation, gradual deterioration (months, years)
conscious state	alert
attention	poor concentration
affect	limited
memory	impaired
thinking	impaired
judgement	impaired
orientation	variably disorientated
hallucinations	rare
speech	stereotyped, limited
insight	often unaware

Assessment. The diagnosis is established by mental state and neuropsychological testing. Early dementia must be distinguished from depression. A diagnosis of depression is suggested by an acute onset, poor self image, guilt, withdrawal and apathy. On examination, the depressed patient can produce answers, whereas the truly demented cannot.

Treatment

General measures. Patients with mild dementia may require no specific treatment unless a secondary acute confusional state develops. Patients with dementia will fare better in familiar surroundings which should be simplified as much as possible to reduce demands on them. They are not kept in hospital unless necessary and their neuropsychiatric condition may improve after discharge home. Patients incapable of self-care need varying amounts of assistance. The condition needs to be explained to the patient and the family and reassurance given that the disorder has an organic basis.

Treatment of cause. A potentially treatable cause (e.g. hydrocephalus, thyroid dysfunction) should always be considered. Treatment of malignant infiltration or central nervous system infection can lead to improvement. There is no specific treatment for the paraneoplastic syndromes.

INSOMNIA

Cause (Table 9.13). Insomnia is frequently multifactorial.

Table 9.13 Causes of insomnia

physical	drug related
pain	drugs causing insomnia
dyspnea, hypoxia, cough	corticosteroids
fevers, sweats, pruritus	amphetamines, methylphenidate, cocaine
nocturia, polyuria	xanthines
diarrhea	caffeine
fear of urinary or fecal incontinence	drug withdrawal causing insomnia
psychological, psychiatric	benzodiazepines
anxiety	barbiturates
depression	alcohol
psychosis, mania	nicotine
acute confusion or delirium	
dementia	
fear of dying	
environmental factors	

Treatment

General measures. Management includes treatment of any physical or psychological factors which may be preventing or disturbing sleep (Table 9.14). Some patients with advanced cancer have a great fear of dying in their sleep and need to discuss these fears and anxieties. Good psychological support and relaxation therapy can be of great benefit. Environmental factors which prevent or disturb sleep such as noise, need for a night light, bed comfort and hospital routines are managed appropriately.

Drug therapy. Temazepam has an intermediate half-life of 8-10 hours and does not produce metabolites which cause cumulative toxicity. The usual dose is 10-20 mg orally. Patients unable to take temazepam can be treated with sublingual lorazepam or subcutaneous midazolam. Patients with insomnia and acute confusion or delirium are treated with chlorpromazine or haloperidol.

Table 9.14 Treatment of insomnia

treat any factors related to physical disease which may be causing or aggravating insomnia
assess the patient's medications
treat any psychological or psychiatric factors which may be causing or aggravating insomnia
control environmental disturbances and discomforts
benzodiazepines e.g. temazepam

PARANEOPLASTIC SYNDROMES

The neurological paraneoplastic syndromes are an uncommon and heterogeneous group of disorders which are remote or nonmetastatic effects of cancer on the nervous system (Table 9.15)

Table 9.15 Paraneoplastic syndromes affecting the nervous system

brain	subacute cerebellar degeneration
	limbic encephalitis
	opsoclonus-myoclonus syndrome
	progressive multifocal leukoencephalopathy
spinal cord	subacute necrotizing myelopathy
	subacute motor neuropathy
peripheral nerve	sensory neuropathy
	sensorimotor polyneuropathy
	ascending acute polyneuropathy (Guillain-Barré syndrome)
	autonomic neuropathy
neuromuscular	myasthenic syndrome (Eaton-Lambert syndrome)
	dermatomyositis, polymyositis (see Ch 7)

Clinical features. The neuropathies, particularly the sensorimotor type, are the only syndromes commonly seen. The paraneoplastic syndromes may precede, follow or coincide with the diagnosis of cancer. In some cases the syndromes run a course independent of the progression (or regression, with treatment) of the primary tumor. Recognition of the neurological paraneoplastic syndromes may allow better explanation of a patient's symptoms.

Treatment. Some of these syndromes respond to anticancer, corticosteroid or immunosuppressive treatment, and specific therapy is available for patients with the myasthenic syndrome (see Chapter 7).

EYE PROBLEMS

Conjunctivitis

Cause. Conjunctivitis is acute inflammation of the conjunctiva due to infection, allergy or other toxic reaction (Table 9.16).

Table 9.16 Conjunctivitis

infection	bacterial
	viral : adenovirus, herpes virus
allergy	
drug reaction	fluorouracil, methotrexate, cytarabine
radiotherapy	acute inflammation
	chronic dryness
loss of blinking	VII nerve palsy, proptosis

Clinical features. There is mild discomfort associated with watering, itching and a gritty feeling in the eye. Vision is well preserved. Examination shows diffuse conjunctival inflammation.

Treatment. The treatment of conjunctivitis is with regular saline washes. If there is significant discharge, suggesting bacterial infection, topical antibiotics can be used. If the condition worsens, bacteriological and viral swabs are taken and ophthalmological opinion sought. Treatment of viral conjunctivitis is symptomatic using washes and topical lubricants and antiviral agents are reserved for corneal disease (see below).

Keratitis

Cause. Keratitis, or inflammation of the cornea, is usually due to infection or to trauma secondary to an inability to close the eye (Table 9.17).

Table 9.17 Keratitis

infection	HSV, VZV
	bacterial
	fungal
traumatic	VIIth nerve palsy, proptosis
radiotherapy	acute inflammation
	chronic dryness
immune	keratoconjunctivitis sicca

Clinical features. Keratitis is characterized by conjunctivitis, pain, photophobia and watering of the eye. There is usually some blurring of vision. Infection with herpes simplex virus (HSV) is usually associated with signs of nasolabial infection and dendritic ulceration is seen on ophthalmological examination. Infection with the varicella zoster virus (VZV) occurs in association with herpes zoster of the ophthalmic nerves and corneal ulceration is seen on examination. Bacterial infection may occur secondary to traumatic keratitis caused by inability to close the eye, as occurs with proptosis or VIIth nerve palsy.

Treatment. Herpetic infection is treated with topical aciclovir and corticosteroid. Bacterial keratitis is treated with appropriate antibiotics. Traumatic keratitis is treated with topical antibiotics and lubricants (artificial tears) and surgical tarsorrhaphy should be considered if the condition is chronic.

Further Reading - see page 111

10 Psychiatric

> depression
> anxiety

DEPRESSION

Incidence. Significant symptoms of depression are reported to occur in about 25% of patients with cancer. The incidence is higher, probably over 50%, in patients with advancing disease, increasing physical disability or troublesome pain.

Diagnosis. The symptoms upon which a diagnosis of depression is made in physically healthy individuals are shown in Table 10.1. In patients with cancer, the significance of the somatic symptoms is questionable as all may be caused by the cancer itself. The somatic symptoms may be considered significant if they are clearly out of proportion to the physical illness. Other criteria which have been advocated include persistent tearfulness, persistent irritability, a sense of hopelessness, perceiving the illness as punishment and a sense of worthlessness or being a burden.

Table 10.1 Symptoms of depression

psychological	depressed mood
	diminished interests or pleasure in activities
	psychomotor agitation or retardation
	lack of concentration or indecision
	diminished self esteem, feelings of guilt
	thoughts of death or suicide
somatic	significant change in appetite and/or weight
	insomnia or hypersomnia
	fatigue and/or loss of energy

Adapted from : Diagnostic and statistical manual of mental disorders, 3rd edition, revised (DSM-III-R). Washington DC. American Psychiatric Association, 1987.

Clinical features. Symptoms of depression can occur as part of the normal response to a crisis, in reactive depression, as part of a major affective illness or in association with an organic brain syndrome (Table 10.2).

Table 10.2 Types of depression seen in patients with cancer

'normal '
    part of transient normal response to crises, stress
adjustment disorder
    reactive depression ± reactive anxiety
major depressive illness
organic brain syndromes
    acute confusional state or delirium
    dementia
    side effect of drugs

'Normal' depression. Episodes of depression and anxiety occur as part of the normal psychological stress response at times of crisis such as treatment failure or disease progression. These reactions last one to two weeks during which significant symptoms of anxiety and depression may occur. They resolve spontaneously with time and appropriate supportive care from family, friends and the treatment team.

Reactive depression. Reactive depression or an adjustment disorder differs from the normal self limited stress response in either degree or duration. The symptoms last longer than expected (more than two weeks) and may be more severe or intense, causing more disruption and interference with daily functioning, social activities and relationships with others. Reactive depression is frequently associated with anxiety and patients may demonstrate an obsessive concern with symptoms.

Major or endogenous depression. Serious depression occurs in a small proportion of patients with advanced cancer. Compared to reactive depression, the symptoms are usually more severe and the mood is incongruent with the disease outlook and does not respond to support, understanding, caring or distraction. Delusional thoughts and hallucinations, features of psychotic depression, are rare except in patients with organic brain syndromes.

Organic brain syndromes. Patients with acute confusional states (delirium) or dementia may exhibit features of depression. Examination of the patient's mental state including memory, concentration and attention, orientation, thinking and comprehension will reveal evidence of organic brain dysfunction. A number of drugs can cause a depressive syndrome.

Assessment. The assessment of depression in patients with cancer depends on the duration and severity of the symptoms and needs to be carried out in the context of the patient's overall illness and prognosis (Table 10.3). Assessment may be aided by patient-administered questionnaires validated for use in patients with cancer, such as the Hospital Anxiety and Depression Scale (HADS) or the Rotterdam Symptoms Checklist (RSCL).

Table 10.3 Assessment of patients with cancer and depression or anxiety

exclude organic brain syndrome
    acute confusional state, dementia, drug side effects
assess the state of physical disease, prognosis
assess other potential causative or aggravating factors
    pain, other physical symptoms, social, cultural, spiritual
assess family and social supports
assess severity of depression or anxiety
assess other psychological factors
    understanding of medical situation
    insight into illness
    impact of illness
    concurrent life stresses
    past losses and how they coped
    history of anxiety or other psychiatric illness
    history of alcoholism, substance abuse

Treatment

Optimal therapy includes supportive counselling and psychotherapy in addition to antidepressant medications. If an organic brain syndrome is present it is treated appropriately (see Chapter 9). Treatment of other problems causing or aggravating depression, particularly pain, can be of great benefit.

'Normal' depression. Patients with normal transient depression occurring in response to acute crises usually require only good general supportive care (Table 10.4). Short term use of a hypnotic at night and an anxiolytic by day is of benefit in severe cases. Psychotherapy is not usually required although relaxation training may be helpful if anxiety is pronounced.

Table 10.4 Treatment of depression

diagnose and treat organic brain syndrome, if present
treat any causative or aggravating factors
pain, other physical symptoms, social, cultural, spiritual
general support
caring and empathy
reassurance of continued care and interest
provision of information about illness
explore patients' understanding and fears about illness, prognosis
encourage, strengthen family and social supports
brief, supportive psychotherapy
clarification and resolution of problems regarding disease, treatment, future, coping, etc.
family, group therapy
behavioral techniques
antidepressants
other drugs : hypnotics, anxiolytics, neuroleptics

Psychotherapy. Patients with more severe depression, reactive or endogenous, require more intensive therapy with both psychotherapy and antidepressants. Psychotherapy should be of short duration (4 to 6 weeks), supportive, and aim for conflict resolution or acceptance. It is directed at clarification and resolution of problems pertaining to the patient's medical situation, the goals and expectations of treatment and fears about suffering and death. It is designed to improve coping skills and previously successful coping mechanisms are reinforced. Behavioral techniques such as relaxation therapy may reduce anxiety and allow the patient to have some sense of being in control. This type of brief psychotherapy should include family members and will provide them with appropriate support as well as a better insight into the patient's problems.

Tricyclic antidepressants. The various tricyclic antidepressants cause varying degrees of sedation, anticholinergic and cardiovascular side effects and different drugs are more suited to certain situations. Patients with agitation or insomnia are treated with a sedating antidepressant such as amitriptyline or doxepin; patients with psychomotor slowing require a less sedating drug such as desipramine, and patients with problems related to intestinal motility or urinary retention need a drug with less anticholinergic effect such as desipramine or nortriptyline. Tricyclic antidepressants are usually started at a dose of 50-100 mg at night and increased gradually over several weeks; most adult patients require doses of 150 mg/d. Side effects are common and can be clinically troublesome, especially in elderly or frail patients.

Other antidepressants. Fluoxetine, paroxetine and sertraline are selective serotonin re-uptake inhibitors (SSRI). They have little sedative, anticholinergic or cardiac side effects but can cause transient anxiety, insomnia, anorexia and weight loss during the first few weeks of treatment. Monoamine oxidase inhibitors (MAOI) should be avoided in patients with advanced cancer because of the need for dietary restrictions and the frequency of interactions with other drugs.

Other drugs. The use of a hypnotic at night and an anxiolytic during the day can be useful adjuvant therapy in depression. Patients with depression and psychotic symptoms or an acute confusional state are treated with haloperidol or chlorpromazine.

ANXIETY

Clinical features. Symptoms of anxiety may occur in different situations in patients with cancer and should be regarded as a continuous clinical spectrum ranging from normal to psychiatric (Table 10.5). The physical symptoms and signs of anxiety are numerous (Table 10.6).

Table 10.5 Types of anxiety

normal
    transient anxiety in response to stress, crises
adjustment disorder
    reactive anxiety ± depression
organic anxiety syndromes
    uncontrolled pain
    hypoxia, respiratory distress
    any uncontrolled or severe physical symptoms
    acute confusional state or delirium
    drug side effects : corticosteroids, metoclopramide, bronchodilators
    drug withdrawal : opioids, barbiturates, benzodiazepines, alcohol, nicotine
anxiety disorder
    generalized anxiety, panic, phobias

Table 10.6 Clinical features of anxiety

cognitive	non-specific fear, fear of dying, fear of 'going crazy'
	poor attention and concentration
cardiovascular	palpitations, tachycardia, systolic hypertension, chest pain
	flushing, sweating
respiratory	breathlessness, hyperventilation
neurological	dizziness, tremor, paresthesias
	restlessness, weakness, exhaustion, insomnia
gastrointestinal	anorexia, indigestion, diarrhea, air swallowing
general	tense, worried, restless, irritable

Normal anxiety. Anxiety occurs normally in response to the stress and crises associated with cancer and its treatment and is more frequent in the terminal phases of the disease.

Adjustment disorder – reactive anxiety. If a patient's anxiety lasts longer than expected (more than 7 to 14 days) and exceeds the level that is regarded as normal and adaptive, they may be classified as having an adjustment disorder with anxious mood. Reactive anxiety follows a defined incident or stress. Depressive symptoms frequently coexist.

Organic anxiety syndromes. Anxiety occurs with any severe or unrelieved physical symptoms, with acute confusion of any cause and as a side effect of drugs (Table 10.5).

Anxiety disorders.   These patients have more severe and disabling symptoms which appear inappropriate or out of proportion to the medical situation. A generalized anxiety disorder is characterized by chronic unrealistic worries with autonomic hyperactivity, apprehension and hypervigilance. Pre-existing phobias may be activated or aggravated. Panic attacks may occur which consist of sudden, unpredictable attacks of intense fear and physical discomfort, usually lasting 15 to 20 minutes.

Assessment.   Anxiety is a normal and universal emotion. As with depression, the distinction of abnormal anxiety in patients with physical illness is poorly defined. The assessment of the anxious patient is outlined in Table 10.3 and needs to be carried out in the context of the patient's overall illness and prognosis.

Treatment

The treatment of anxiety needs to be an integral part of an overall plan of management for the patient (Table 10.7). The control of pain and other causative or aggravating factors is of particular importance.

Table 10.7   Treatment of anxiety in patients with cancer

treat the cause of organic anxiety syndrome, if present
treat other factors which may cause or aggravate anxiety
pain, other physical symptoms, social, cultural, spiritual
treat depression, if present
general support
brief, supportive psychotherapy
behavioral - relaxation
drug therapy
anxiolytics : benzodiazepines, hydroxyzine, buspirone
other : hypnotics, antidepressants, neuroleptics

Normal anxiety.   Patients with normal anxiety responses do not require special therapy except for good supportive care. Temporary use of a hypnotic at night and an anxiolytic by day is appropriate if the symptoms are severe.

More severe anxiety.   Patients with more severe reactive anxiety benefit from treatment with hypnotics and anxiolytics. Depression is frequently present and the use of antidepressants can be considered. Brief supportive psychotherapy aimed at clarification of anxiety-provoking issues is frequently beneficial. Behavioral techniques including distraction, relaxation therapy (isometric and deep breathing) and stress management techniques will help some patients and may give them a sense of being in control. Hypnosis helps some patients. Treatment is frequently by a combination of anxiolytic medication, supportive counselling and behavioral and relaxation therapy.

Benzodiazepines.   Benzodiazepines are the drugs used most frequently to treat anxiety (Table 10.8). Drugs with short and intermediate half-lives (alprazolam, lorazepam, oxazepam) are preferred to longer acting drugs such as diazepam. Lorazepam can be given sublingually and midazolam as a continuous subcutaneous infusion. The side effects of benzodiazepines include drowsiness, inco-ordination and confusion which are dose related and reversible.

Other anxiolytics.   The antihistamine hydroxyzine has anxiolytic properties and can be given orally or by subcutaneous infusion; the main side effect is sedation. The non-benzodiazepine drug, buspirone, has been shown to be effective in the treatment of anxiety and does not cause significant sedation, but takes 5 to 10 days to be effective.

Table 10.8 Anxiolytic drugs

benzodiazepines			
short acting	:	alprazolam	0.25-0.5 mg PO q4-8h
		midazolam	2-5 mg IM or SC q1-2h or by SC infusion
intermediate	:	lorazepam	1-2 mg PO or SL q6-8h
		oxazepam	15-30 mg PO q8-12h
long acting	:	diazepam	5-10 mg PO q8-12h
antihistamine		hydroxyzine	25-50 mg PO q8-12h or by SC infusion
other		buspirone	5-10 mg PO q8h

Other drugs. A hypnotic such as temazepam is often helpful in the management of anxiety. Antidepressants can be used if there is coexistent depression. Haloperidol or chlorpromazine are indicated for severe anxiety or agitation not controlled with a benzodiazepine and in patients with psychotic features or acute confusional states.

Further Reading - see page 111

11 Endocrine and metabolic

> hypercalcemia
> hypernatremia and diabetes insipidus
> hyponatremia and SIADH
> hypokalemia and ectopic ACTH
>
> hypoglycemia
> carcinoid syndrome
> islet cell carcinomas
> gynecomastia

HYPERCALCEMIA

Cause. In the majority of patients with solid tumors, hypercalcemia is due to secretion of parathyroid hormone-related protein (PTHrP) by the tumor. PTHrP stimulates osteoclastic bone resorption with mobilization of skeletal calcium and explains hypercalcemia in patients with no bone metastases. Hypercalcemia may also occur with local bone destruction in which a range of cytokines produced by tumor cells activate osteoclasts. Treatment of breast cancer with tamoxifen or other hormonal therapy can produce a 'flare' reaction with hypercalcemia and increased bone pain; the mechanism is uncertain but possibly relates to prostaglandins. A number of other factors, unrelated to the tumor, can also cause or predispose to hypercalcemia (Table 11.1).

Table 11.1 Hypercalcemia : etiology

associated with cancer	*not due to cancer*
humoral (PTHrP)	immobilization
bone destruction	excess ingestion of calcium, vitamins A or D
tamoxifen or other hormonal therapy	milk alkali syndrome
	thiazide diuretics
	primary hyperparathyroidism

Clinical features (Table 11.2). The severity of the symptoms depends on the level of (nonprotein-bound) ionized calcium and the speed with which the level rises. Coexistent acidosis increases the ionized calcium level and can precipitate symptoms; alkalosis has the opposite effect.

Table 11.2 Clinical features of hypercalcemia

gastrointestinal	anorexia, nausea and vomiting, constipation, abdominal pain
renal	polyuria, nocturia, polydipsia, dehydration
neurological	tiredness, weakness, apathy, irritability, confusion, drowsiness, coma
other	increased bone pain, pruritus

Treatment

All patients symptomatic of hypercalcemia warrant a trial of therapy; bisphosphonate therapy is effective in the majority of patients and is relatively free of side effects.

General measures. A number of general measures are useful in the treatment of mild hypercalcemia or in the maintenance of normocalcemia after bisphosphonate therapy (Table 11.3). Low calcium diets probably have no effect on malignant hypercalcemia.

Table 11.3 Hypercalcemia : general measures

maintain mobility, avoid immobilization
increased fluid intake – 3 l/d
stop thiazide diuretics
dietary
    stop calcium or vitamin supplements, excess milk or antacids
    normal calcium diet
treatment of underlying disease, where possible and appropriate
    radiotherapy, hormonal therapy, chemotherapy

Rehydration. The treatment of severe hypercalcemia is initially by intravenous rehydration with normal saline (Table 11.4). The addition of furosemide may increase calcium excretion but should not be used until the patient is fully rehydrated.

Bisphosphonates.   The bisphosphonates are chemical analogues of pyrophosphate and inhibit bone resorption. Pamidronate is more effective and has a longer duration of action than other bisphosphonate compounds. The effect is usually evident within 1 to 2 days but, unless treatment has been given to control the underlying disease, further therapy is often required within 2 to 4 weeks. Repeated therapy may produce lesser responses. Mild nausea and fever are the only frequently reported side effects of pamidronate.   Oral etidronate can be used for the maintenance of normocalcemia.

Other drugs. Calcitonin is used for the rapid correction of severe hypercalcemia but continued injections are required and it may cause nausea and vomiting. Oral phosphate (1-3 g/d) acts by raising the serum phosphate level, causing a secondary lowering of the serum calcium; it cannot be used in patients with renal failure or hyperphosphatemia. Its main side effect is diarrhea which is dose-limiting and a frequent cause for patient noncompliance. Corticosteroids are frequently advocated in the treatment of hypercalcemia but are only of use in corticosteroid-sensitive tumors including myeloma, lymphoma and some patients with breast and prostate cancer. Treatment is started at a higher dose, such as prednisolone 50 mg/day, and tapered according to response.

Table 11.4 Hypercalcemia : drug therapy

rehydration with normal saline ± furosemide
bisphosphonate : pamidronate 30-90 mg IV in 500 ml normal saline over 2-3h
calcitonin 100-200 units IM, SC q12h
oral phosphate
corticosteroids

HYPERNATREMIA AND DIABETES INSIPIDUS

Cause. Hypernatremia may result from either inadequate fluid intake or increased fluid losses (Table 11.5). Diabetes insipidus is caused by deficient secretion of antidiuretic hormone (ADH) by the pituitary gland due to primary or secondary infiltration of the pituitary or hypothalamus.

Clinical features. The significant clinical features of diabetes insipidus relate to cerebral dehydration which progressively causes lethargy, weakness, restlessness, irritability, muscle twitching, seizures, coma and death.

Table 11.5 Causes of hypernatremia

decreased fluid intake (relative or absolute)
bedridden, semiconscious, aphagia
increased fluid loss
gastrointestinal: vomiting, diarrhea, fistulas, nasogastric drainage
renal : diuretic therapy, hyperglycemia
: diuresis following renal failure or obstruction
: diabetes insipidus
skin : fever, sweating, hot environment
pulmonary : hyperventilation, dry atmosphere
third space fluid collection : bowel obstruction, ascites

Assessment. The diagnosis is made by the measurement of the serum sodium level and the serum and urine osmolality. The blood osmolality will be elevated above 280 mmol/kg and the urine osmolality rarely exceeds 200 mmol/kg.

Treatment

General measures. Treatment consists of repletion of total body water, matching any continuing losses and treating the underlying cause. Body water needs to be replaced gradually to avoid cerebral edema.

Hormonal therapy. Diabetes insipidus is treated by hormone replacement with vasopressin (the natural human hormone, made synthetically) or desmopressin (a synthetic analogue with a longer duration of action). Initial therapy for a seriously ill patient is usually with vasopressin which can be given intramuscularly or subcutaneously. The dose is 5 to 10 units and subsequent doses can be given after 6 to 8 hours if polyuria recurs. Continuing therapy is with intranasal desmopressin, 10-40 µg/d intranasally, given as two divided doses.

HYPONATREMIA AND SIADH

Causes of hyponatremia are listed in Table 11.6. Clinical assessment will usually define the cause, to which treatment is directed.

Table 11.6 Causes of hyponatremia

pseudohyponatremia	
paraproteinemia : myeloma, macroglobulinemia	
hyperglycemia	
excess water drinking	
edematous states	
cardiac, renal, hepatic failure	
hypothyroidism	
salt wasting states	
mineralocorticoid or corticosteroid deficiency, diuretics, chronic renal failure	
gastrointestinal losses (without adequate sodium replacement)	
vomiting, diarrhea, fistulas	
excess ADH for diabetes insipidus	
syndrome of inappropriate ADH	
tumors	small cell lung cancer, others
neurological	primary or metastatic tumor, post neurosurgery
pulmonary	pneumonia, abscess, TB
drugs	vincristine, cyclophosphamide, carbamazepine, chlorpropamide, thiazides

Syndrome of inappropriate antidiuretic hormone secretion (SIADH)

Cause. This syndrome is characterized by the excessive and inappropriate secretion of antidiuretic hormone (ADH) either by a tumor or as the result of other influences acting on the posterior pituitary gland (Table 11.6). In SIADH there is reduced renal excretion of water, leading to a state of water intoxication with hyponatremia and hypotonicity of the plasma.

Clinical features. The signs and symptoms of SIADH depend on the severity of the hyponatremia and the rapidity of onset. Symptoms are uncommon until the serum sodium falls below 125 mmol/l or the plasma osmolality (P_{osm}) below 250 mmol/kg. The initial symptoms are nonspecific and include anorexia, nausea and general malaise. With progressive hyponatremia and hypotonicity, signs and symptoms of cerebral edema develop with headache, lethargy, confusion and agitation, leading to obtundation, seizures and coma which can be fatal.

Assessment. The diagnosis of SIADH is made on the basis of a low serum sodium, low plasma osmolality (P_{osm} <270 mmol/kg), and a urine osmolality reflecting inappropriately concentrated urine (U_{osm} usually >500 mmol/kg). Other conditions may occasionally produce a similar picture and it is customary to exclude the presence of dehydration or hepatic, cardiac, renal, adrenal and thyroid dysfunction.

Treatment. Mild cases usually respond well to fluid restriction. The underlying cause is treated, where possible and appropriate. The antibiotic, demeclocycline, is useful when fluid restriction is otherwise undesirable and for patients whose cancer is unlikely to respond to anticancer therapy. More severe SIADH requires special management of fluids (Table 11.7).

Table 11.7 Management of SIADH

correct or treat cause, where possible
demeclocycline 300-600 mg PO q12h
management of fluids

se Na >120 mmol/l and asymptomatic
fluid restriction : 500-1000 ml/d

se Na 110-120 mmol/l without serious symptoms
fluid restriction : 500 ml/d
furosemide 40-80 mg PO or IV q6h
replacement of urinary electrolyte losses (IV saline)

se Na <110 mmol/l or serious symptoms
3% hypertonic saline 1 l q6-8h
furosemide 40-80 mg IV q6-8h
cardiac failure : additional furosemide
  decrease infusion rate
neurological deterioration : dexamethasone 4-20 mg IV
  mannitol 25-50 g IV

HYPOKALEMIA AND ECTOPIC ACTH

Causes of hypokalemia relevant to patients with advanced cancer are shown in Table 11.8. Hypokalemia causes muscle weakness and cramps, constipation and paralytic ileus, and predisposes to cardiac arrhythmias. Treatment is with oral or parenteral supplements in addition to therapy directed at the underlying cause.

Table 11.8 Causes of hypokalemia

inadequate intake, malnutrition	hormonal
gastrointestinal losses	mineralocorticoid excess
vomiting, nasogastric drainage	hyperaldosteronism
intestinal fistulas, diarrhea	mineralocorticoid administration
chronic laxative abuse	corticosteroid excess
renal losses	Cushing's syndrome
diuretics	ectopic ACTH production
osmotic diuresis (hyperglycemia)	corticosteroid administration
antibiotics, corticosteroids	

Ectopic ACTH

Cause. The secretion of adrenocorticotrophic hormone (ACTH) by tumors will cause excess cortisone secretion by the adrenal gland, leading to a type of Cushing's syndrome. Ectopic ACTH secretion is characteristically associated with small cell carcinoma of the lung and less frequently with other tumors.

Clinical features. Ectopic ACTH secretion causes hypokalemia, profound muscle weakness, hyperglycemia, weight loss and edema. The characteristic physical features of Cushing's syndrome are usually absent.

Diagnosis. The diagnosis of ectopic ACTH production is made on the findings of hypokalemic alkalosis, increased cortisol levels without diurnal variation, and increased levels of ACTH which do not suppress with dexamethasone administration.

Treatment. Treatment is primarily directed at the underlying tumor. If the tumor is not amenable to therapy, or while such treatment is being initiated, the use of a drug which suppresses adrenal function (aminoglutethimide 250 mg, 3 or 4 times daily) can be of value. If complete adrenal suppression is achieved, the patient will require corticosteroid replacement at physiological dosage. Ectopic ACTH production can occasionally be inhibited by the somatostatin analogue, octreotide.

HYPOGLYCEMIA

Cause (Table 11.9). Tumor-related hypoglycemia is due to insulin-like growth factors produced by the tumors.

Table 11.9 Causes of hypoglycemia

starvation
excess insulin : iatrogenic, insulinomas
tumor related hypoglycemia : soft tissue sarcomas, mesotheliomas, hepatomas
extensive liver metastases

Clinical features. Hypoglycemic attacks may be heralded by tremor, hunger and sweating. More commonly, they present with weakness, fatigue, dizziness, confusion and somnolence. Seizures and coma can occur in severe cases.

Treatment. Treatment of tumor-related hypoglycemia is primarily directed at the tumor. Symptomatic management involves the regular ingestion of food or sugar. In severe or resistant cases, therapy with corticosteroids can be tried. Diazoxide, which inhibits insulin secretion, is used for patients with insulinomas.

CARCINOID SYNDROME

Cause. Carcinoid tumors occur most frequently in the ileum and appendix with a small proportion in the colon and rectum; about 10% of primary carcinoid tumors are pulmonary. When hepatic metastases develop and tumor products are released into the systemic circulation, the carcinoid syndrome occurs.

Clinical features. The carcinoid syndrome comprises cutaneous flushing, diarrhea, wheezing and right heart failure. The metabolic symptoms are caused by serotonin as well as a host of other substances released from the tumors including kallikrein, substance P and other neuropeptides, prostaglandins, histamine and catecholamines. Pulmonary carcinoid tumors may also secrete ACTH and ADH.

Treatment

Therapy of the carcinoid syndrome (Table 11.10) includes standard therapy for diarrhea and bronchospasm.

Antiserotonin agents. Various antiserotonin agents are used to treat the flushing and diarrhea. They are effective for a proportion of patients, the response rate being greater with milder disease.

Octreotide. The somatostatin analogue, octreotide, will reduce flushing and diarrhea for more than 80% of patients. The duration of response is uncertain and, when symptoms recur, increasing the dose is sometimes effective. The only common side effect is transient pain at the injection site. Insulin-dependent diabetics may require less insulin.

Ondansetron. The $5HT_3$ receptor antagonist, ondansetron, is also reported to be effective against the flushing and diarrhea of the carcinoid syndrome.

Carcinoid crisis. Carcinoid crisis is a potentially life threatening event which occurs in patients with the carcinoid syndrome, usually associated with stress such as general anesthesia. There is a severe and persistent flush associated with abdominal pain and an exacerbation of diarrhea. There can be severe hypotension or hypertension and CNS depression. Intravenous octreotide usually reverses this syndrome promptly; it is not known whether pretreatment with octreotide prevents its occurrence.

Table 11.10 Treatment of carcinoid syndrome

standard therapy
    diarrhea : loperamide, codeine
    bronchospasm : albuterol
antiserotonin agents
    cyproheptadine 4 mg PO q8h
    chlorpheniramine 4 mg PO q8h + cimetidine 400 mg PO q12h
octreotide 0.05 mg SC q12h, and titrate
ondansetron 8 mg PO q8h

ISLET CELL CARCINOMAS

Pancreatic islet cell carcinomas are rare tumors which produce a range of active hormonal substances (Table 11.11) and a variety of different clinical syndromes.

Treatment. Insulinomas may be treated with diazoxide which inhibits the release of insulin; octreotide therapy is successful in a proportion of patients. The Zollinger-Ellison syndrome is treated with high doses of H_2-receptor antagonists or omeprazole. Octreotide is frequently effective with tumors secreting glucagon or vasoactive intestinal polypeptides (VIP), although the responses may not be durable. The treatment of the other syndromes listed are dealt with elsewhere in this chapter.

Table 11.11 Clinical features of pancreatic islet cell carcinomas

Hormone	Clinical syndrome
insulin	hypoglycemia
gastrin	Zollinger-Ellison syndrome (abdominal pain, severe peptic ulcer disease)
glucagon	diabetes, rash, muscle weakness
vasoactive intestinal polypeptide	watery diarrhea
parathyroid hormone	hypercalcemia
serotonin	carcinoid syndrome
adrenocorticotrophic hormone	ectopic ACTH syndrome
antidiuretic hormone	SIADH

GYNECOMASTIA

Cause (Table 11.12). Gynecomastia in men is caused by a deficiency of androgens or a relative or absolute excess of estrogens.

Treatment. Medications thought to be causing gynecomastia should be stopped, if possible. Otherwise, treatment is by reassurance.

Table 11.12 Gynecomastia

diminished androgen	drugs (various mechanisms)
orchidectomy	digoxin
decreased synthesis	spironolactone
old age	cimetidine
estrogens, progestogens, LHRH analogues	ketoconazole
decreased action : flutamide, cyproterone acetate	antidepressants
increased estrogen	antihypertensives
estrogen therapy	phenothiazines
estrogen secreting tumors	
gonadotrophin secreting tumors	
germ cell tumors : testicular, extra-testicular	
lung cancer, other tumors	
liver disease	

Further Reading - see page 111

12 Constitutional

> anorexia   dehydration
> cachexia   fevers and sweats
> asthenia   hormonal flushes

ANOREXIA

Anorexia is a reduced desire to eat.

Cause (Table 12.1). Patients with advanced cancer frequently have multiple causes.

Table 12.1 Causes of anorexia

cancer	
pain	
intracranial disease	metastases, radiotherapy
disordered taste, smell	cancer
	stomatitis
	malodorous ulcer or fungating tumor
	radiotherapy, chemotherapy, other drugs
gastrointestinal	stomatitis
	esophagitis, dysphagia
	small stomach : gastrectomy, linitis plastica
	gastric compression : hepatomegaly, splenomegaly, ascites
	gastric distension, delayed gastric emptying
	bowel obstruction, constipation
	hepatic metastases
metabolic	abnormalities of sodium, calcium, sugar
	organ failure : liver, kidney, adrenal
infections	
drugs	
psychological	anxiety, depression, disinterest
	intolerance of institutional food, unappetizing food
religious or cultural customs	

Treatment

Treatment of anorexia is important as it will improve patient morale, reduce family anxiety and the preservation of optimal nutrition may delay the onset of cachexia. The primary treatment of anorexia is that of the cause and many of the listed causes are amenable to some degree of palliation. The assistance of a dietician may be invaluable.

Appetite stimulants. The use of appetite stimulants (Table 12.2) can be of benefit but, with the possible exception of progestogens, have little effect on objective measures of nutritional status or the development of cachexia. A small amount of alcohol taken before or with meals may stimulate appetite as well as improving mood and providing a few calories. Corticosteroids will produce subjective improvement in appetite and well-being in the majority of patients, although the effect may last only a few weeks. The dose can be doubled if there is no response or when the initial response wanes. Treatment with a progestogen leads to improved appetite, weight gain and improvement in subjective well being. Side effects include fluid retention, hypertension and thrombophlebitis.

Table 12.2 Management of anorexia

treat or palliate the underlying cause
activity, exercise
dietary
    dietary advice (dietician)
    small frequent meals
    what they want, when they want it
    tasty, visually appealing food
    eat sitting at a table, in a room free of odors
appetite stimulants
    alcohol
    corticosteroids : prednisolone 15-30 mg/d
    progestogens : megestrol 160 mg/d *or* medroxyprogesterone 400 mg/d
explanation, counselling

Counselling. Anorexia and poor nutritional intake frequently cause much distress for patients and families and require careful discussion and explanation. When advanced and progressing cancer is the prime cause, it needs to be explained that enteral or parenteral nutrition will be of no benefit.

CACHEXIA

Cachexia is progressive wasting caused by metabolic alterations associated with advancing cancer.

Cause. The cachexia of advanced cancer is primarily due to alterations in protein, carbohydrate and lipid metabolism caused by inflammatory cytokines released by the tumor (Table 12.3). The role of nutrition is minor and cachexia cannot be prevented by enteral and parenteral nutrition. The nutritional requirements of the tumor also make a minor contribution.

Clinical features. The clinical features of cachexia are well known (Table 12.4).

Table 12.3 Causes of cachexia

metabolic abnormalities due to presence of tumor
malnutrition
    poor intake due to anorexia (see Table 12.1)
    functional blockage : mouth, esophagus, stomach
    malabsorption
    vomiting, diarrhea, fistulas
    protein loss : ulceration, hemorrhage, repeated paracenteses
    general effects of surgery, radiotherapy, chemotherapy
tumor metabolism

Table 12.4 Clinical features of cachexia

weight loss	pallor, anemia
lethargy	edema (hypoalbuminemia)
muscle wasting, asthenia	poor wound healing
loss of body fat	pressure sores

Treatment

The treatment options are listed in Table 12.5.

Table 12.5 Treatment of cachexia

correct or palliate cause of malnutrition, anorexia
treat tumor, where feasible
drug treatment of cachexia
dietary measures
    general measures
    dietary supplements
    enteral nutrition
    parenteral nutrition
management of the psychosocial consequences

Drug therapy. There is no satisfactory drug therapy for cachexia. Corticosteroids, cyproheptadine, alcohol and metoclopramide may reduce anorexia but have no effect on the metabolic abnormalities of cachexia. The progestogens may exert an anabolic effect, increasing lean body mass and fat, but an effect on survival has not been demonstrated.

Dietary. Dietary and nutritional therapy may improve a patient's psychological state and reduce family anxieties. A patient will feel more cared for if concern is expressed about nutritional intake and dietary advice given. General measures include providing small frequent meals, of what the patients want and when they want it. Liquid nutritional supplements containing most of the dietary requirements of protein and carbohydrate are commercially available. The use of a multivitamin supplement will do no harm and may be appreciated by the patient and family.

Enteral feeding. Enteral feeding with a nasogastric tube or gastrostomy has little place in the management of patients with advanced cancer. With the exception of patients with upper gastrointestinal obstruction (who may otherwise suffer starvation), enteral feeding will not reverse or prevent cachexia. The side effects of enteral feeding include fluid overload, abdominal cramps and diarrhea.

Parenteral nutrition. For patients with advanced cancer, total parenteral nutrition (TPN) is not effective in improving either survival or the response to anticancer treatment and is associated with significant complications and cost. The exception is a patient who will be temporarily unable to eat for two weeks or more because of anticancer treatment, for whom TPN would be appropriate.

Counselling. The compassionate management of the psychological and social consequences of cachexia is difficult but important. For both the patient and the family, progressive cachexia represents progression of the cancer and counselling and discussions may facilitate acceptance and understanding. The family need to be dissuaded from trying to force the patient to eat, as this will only cause physical distress and guilt. They need to be helped to show love to the patient by means other than feeding them or pressuring them to eat.

ASTHENIA : WEAKNESS AND FATIGUE

Asthenia is generalized weakness associated with fatigue and lassitude.

Cause. Asthenia is most frequently associated with progression of the cancer although other causes need to be considered as some are amenable to treatment or palliation (Table 12.6).

Table 12.6 Causes of generalized weakness and asthenia

neuromuscular	cachexia-related loss of muscle mass
	cachexia-related muscular dysfunction
	myasthenic syndrome (Eaton-Lambert)
	polymyositis
	overactivity, prolonged immobility
	polyneuropathy : carcinomatous or independent of cancer
	intracranial tumor, paraneoplastic encephalopathies
	acute confusion or delirium
metabolic	electrolyte imbalance, dehydration
	renal, hepatic failure
endocrine	adrenal insufficiency, ectopic ACTH secretion, diabetes
malnutrition	inanition, malabsorption
anemia	
infection	
psychological	anxiety, depression, dependency, boredom, insomnia
anticancer therapy	radiotherapy, chemotherapy, interferon
drugs	opioids, tranquillizers, sedatives, antidepressants
	diuretics, antihypertensives, hypoglycemics

Treatment

Treatment of the underlying cause. Treatment is that of the cause, where possible. Correction of some of the uncommon metabolic disturbances listed in Table 12.6 may lead to significant improvement. Transfusion will be of benefit if the patient is severely anemic but the response is often suboptimal and transient.

Drug therapy. Corticosteroids will provide symptomatic improvement in the majority of patients although the effect may last only a few weeks. Corticosteroids should be used with care because of the risk of proximal myopathy with continued therapy. Amphetamines and methylphenidate are also reported to produce symptomatic improvement.

Counselling. For most patients, progressive weakness is a reflection of advancing disease and there are no correctable or treatable underlying causes. Management consists of physical and psychological supportive therapy to enable patients to adjust and cope as well as possible. Psychological adaptation to progressive weakness is the more difficult and the patient and family may have to redefine goals and expectations.

DEHYDRATION

Patients not terminally ill. Parenteral hydration is warranted for symptoms or signs of dehydration in patients unable to take or retain adequate fluids.

Terminally ill patients. Whether or not terminally ill patients benefit from intravenous or subcutaneous fluid administration is controversial. Decisions have to be individualized and depend very much on how close the patient is to death. A bedridden patient will not suffer the weakness and postural hypotension experienced by a patient still ambulatory.

Proponents of artificial hydration claim dehydration causes a dry mouth, thirst and diminished conscious state. However, there are reports (in which some patients received intravenous or subcutaneous hydration) which show no correlation between the state of hydration/dehydration and these symptoms. Dying patients do not complain of thirst and a dry mouth is well palliated with topical therapy.

Alternatively, it can be argued that dehydration occurs normally as part of the dying process and may be of benefit. Reduced urine output requires less movement needed to void and incontinence is less likely; less gastrointestinal secretions can reduce nausea, vomiting and diarrhea; less respiratory secretions reduce dyspnea and terminal congestion; edema and effusions may be less troublesome and reduced edema around tumors may aid pain control. Artificial hydration may have the opposite effect and worsen the patient's situation.

FEVERS AND SWEATS

Cause (Table 12.7). Tumor-related fever is due to the release of pyrogens which act on the temperature regulating centre in the hypothalamus.

Table 12.7   Causes of fever and sweats

infection
cancer
environmental factors
drug reactions
transfusion reactions

Treatment. Treatment is that of the cause, where possible. Control of disease-related fever is best achieved by control of the tumor. If this is not feasible, treatment with one of the NSAIDs is effective in some patients. If refractory and distressing, treatment with corticosteroids (prednisolone 15-30 mg/d) can be tried.

HORMONAL OR HOT FLUSHES

Causes. Hot flushes occur in most women with ovarian failure of whatever cause. Similar symptoms occur in men treated with estrogens, LHRH analogues or by orchidectomy; they are uncommon with antiandrogen therapy.

Clinical features. Hot flushes are described as starting with a discomfort in the lower abdomen or epigastrium, followed quickly by an intense hot feeling ascending towards the head. There is redness of the skin and sweating, often involving the face and head. The episode is short lived and may be followed by a feeling of exhaustion. Hot flushes can be precipitated by emotional upset, hot drinks and meals, a warm room or bed, and alcohol.

Treatment. Treatment in women should be by hormonal replacement with estrogen combined with a progesterone. If estrogen therapy is poorly tolerated or there is an estrogen sensitive tumor, treatment is with a progestogen such as megestrol acetate, 20 mg twice daily or medroxyprogesterone acetate 30-100 mg/d. Clonidine 25-75 µg/d is an alternative but is effective in only a minority of patients. Men are treated with a progestogen, such as megestrol acetate, 20 mg twice daily.

Further Reading - see page 111

Selected Further Reading

Textbooks of Palliative Medicine

Doyle D, Hanks G and MacDonald N (eds). *The Oxford Textbook of Palliative Medicine.* 2nd Edition. Oxford University Press, 1997.

Saunders C and Sykes N (eds). *The Management of Terminal Malignant Disease.* Edward Arnold, 1994.

Twycross R. *Symptom Management in Advanced Cancer.* Radcliffe, 1995

Woodruff R. *Palliative Medicine - Symptomatic and supportive care for patients with advanced cancer and AIDS.* 2nd Edition, Asperula, Melbourne 1996.

Journals

Many articles regarding various aspects of symptom control have been published in general medical and nursing journals. Journals specialising in this field include:

American Journal of Hospice and Palliative Care
European Journal of Palliative Care
International Journal of Palliative Nursing
Journal of Pain and Symptom Management
Palliative Medicine
Progress in Palliative Care
Supportive Care in Cancer

The following lists are a selection of recent articles and reviews.

General

De Vita VT *et al* (eds). *Cancer : Principles and Practice of Oncology.* Lippincott-Raven1997.

Respiratory

Bruera E *et al.* Effects of oxygen on dyspnoea in hypoxaemic terminal cancer patients. *Lancet* 1993; 342 : 13-14.

Bruera E *et al.* Subcutaneous morphine for dyspnoea in cancer patients. *Ann Int Med* 1993; 119 : 906-7.

Davis CL. The role of nebulised drugs in palliating respiratory symptoms of malignant disease. *Eur J Palliative Care* 1995; 2 : 9-15.

Horn LW. Terminal dyspnoea : a hospice approach. *Am J Hospice Palliative Care* 1992; 9 : 24-32.

Petrou M *et al.* Management of recurrent malignant effusions. *Cancer* 1995; 75 : 801-5.

Ruckdeschel JC. Management of malignant pleural effusions. *Sem Oncol* 1995; 22 : Suppl 3, pp 58-63.

Walsh D. Dyspnoea in advanced cancer. *Lancet* 1993; 342 : 450-1.

Gastrointestinal

Alexander-Williams J. Advanced rectal cancer. *BMJ* 1990; 300 : 276-7.

Boyce HW. Stents for palliation of dysphagia due to esophageal cancer. *N Engl J Med* 1992; 329 : 1345-6.

Chambers MS *et al.* Oral and dental management of the cancer patient. *Support Care Cancer* 1995; 3 : 168-75.

Fainsinger RL *et al.* Symptom control in terminally ill patients with malignant bowel obstruction (MBO). *J Pain Symptom Manage* 1994; 9 :12-18.

Forgacs I *et al.* Percutaneous endoscopic gastrostomy. *BMJ* 1992; 304 : 1395-6.

Gough IR and Balderson GA. Malignant ascites. A comparison of peritoneovenous shunting and nonoperative management. *Cancer* 1993; 71 : 2377-82.

Madoff RD *et al.* Fecal incontinence. *N Engl J Med* 1992; 326 : 1002-7.

Mercadante S. Diarrhea in terminally ill patients : pathophysiology and treatment. *J Pain Symptom Manage* 1995; 10 : 298-309.

Raderer M *et al.* Ondansetron for pruritus due to cholestasis. *N Engl J Med* 1994; 330 : 1540.

Regnard C and Cormisky M. Nausea and vomiting in advanced cancer. *Palliative Med* 1992; 6 : 146-51.

Riley J and Fallon MT. Octreotide in terminal malignant obstruction of the gastrointestinal tract. *Eur J Palliative Care* 1994; 1 : 23-6.

Ripamonti C. Management of bowel obstruction in advanced cancer patients. *J Pain Symptom Manage* 1994; 9 : 193-200.

Sharma S and Walsh D. Management of symptomatic malignant ascites with diuretics. *J Pain Symptom Manage* 1995; 10 : 237-42.

Smith AC *et al*. Randomised trial of endoscopic stenting versus surgical bypass in malignant low bile duct obstruction. *Lancet* 1994; 344 : 1655-60.

Soll AH. Pathogenesis of peptic ulcer and implications for therapy. *N Engl J Med* 1990; 322 : 909-16.

Sykes N. The current management of constipation in palliative care. *Prog Palliat Care* 1996; 4 : 170-7

Twycross R. The use of prokinetic drugs in palliative care. *Eur J Palliative Care* 1995; 2 : 143-5.

Genitourinary

De Vries CR and Freiha FS. Haemorrhagic cystitis : a review. *J Urol* 1990; 143 : 1-9.

Greenfield A and Resnick MI. Genitourinary emergencies. *Sem Oncol* 1989; 16 : 516-20.

Regnard C and Mannix K. Urinary problems in advanced cancer - a flow diagram. *Palliative Med* 1991; 5 : 344-8.

Resnick NM. Urinary incontinence. *Lancet* 1995; 346 : 94-9.

Cardiovascular

Badger C and Regnard C. Oedema in advanced disease - a flow diagram. *Palliative Med* 1989; 3 : 213-5.

Bunce IH *et al*. Post-mastectomy lymphoedema treatment and measurement. *Med J Aust* 1994; 161 : 125-8.

Helmes SR and Carlson MD. Cardiovascular emergencies. *Sem Oncol* 1989; 16 : 463-70.

Keane D and Jackson G. Managing recurrent malignant pericardial effusions. *BMJ* 1992; 305 : 729-30.

Wilkes JD *et al*. Malignancy-related pericardial effusion. *Cancer* 1995; 76 : 1377-87.

Hematological

Beutler E *et al* (eds) : *Williams Haematology,* 4th edition. New York, McGraw-Hill, 1995.

Naschitz JE *et al*. Thromboembolism and cancer. *Cancer* 1993; 71 : 1384-90.

Patterson WP (ed) : Coagulation and cancer. *Sem Oncol* 1990; 17 : 137-241.

Schafer AI. Low molecular weight heparin - an opportunity for home treatment of venous thrombosis. *N Engl J Med* 1996; 334 : 724-5.

Schwarz RE et al. Inferior vena cava filters in cancer patients : indications and outcome. *J Clin Oncol* 1996; 14 : 652-657.

Musculoskeletal

Coleman R *et al*. New roles for bisphosphonates in cancer therapy. *Prog Palliat Care* 1996; 4 : 39-43

McEvoy KM *et al*. 3,4-Diaminopyridine in the treatment of Lambert-Eaton myasthenic syndrome. *N Engl J Med* 1989; 321 : 1567-71.

Needham PR and Hoskin PJ. Radiotherapy for painful bone metastases. *Palliative Med* 1994; 8 : 95-104.

Nielsen OS *et al*. Bone metastases : pathophysiology and management policy. *J Clin Oncol* 1991; 9 : 509-24.

Porter AT and Chrisholm GD (eds): Palliation of pain in bony metastases. *Sem Oncol* 1993; 20, Suppl 2 : 1-55.

Siegal T. Muscle cramps in the cancer patient : causes and treatment. *J Pain Symptom Manage* 1991; 6 : 84-91.

Dermatological

Allman RM. Pressure ulcers among the elderly. *N Engl J Med* 1989; 320 : 850-3.

Bale S and Regnard C. Pressure sores in advanced disease : a flow diagram. *Palliative Med* 1989; 3 : 263-5.

De Conno F *et al.* Skin problems in advanced and terminal cancer patients. *J Pain Symptom Manage* 1991; 6 : 247-56.

Editorial : Management of smelly tumours. *Lancet* 1990; 335 : 141-2.

Gilden DH. Herpes zoster with postherpetic neuralgia - persisting pain and frustration. *N Engl J Med* 1994; 330 : 932-4.

Greaves MW. Itching – research has barely scratched the surface. *N Engl J Med* 1992; 326 : 1016-7

Ivetic O and Lyne PA. Fungating and ulcerating malignant lesions. *J Adv Nurs* 1990; 15 : 83-8.

Raderer M *et al.* Ondansetron for pruritus due to cholestasis. *N Engl J Med* 1994; 330 : 1540.

Neurological

Back IN. Terminal restlessness in patients with advanced malignant disease. *Palliative Med* 1992; 6 : 293-8.

Burke A *et al.* Terminal restlessness - its management and the role of midazolam. *Med J Aust* 1991; 155 : 485-7.

Byrne TN. Spinal cord compression from epidural metastases. *N Engl J Med* 1992; 327 : 614-9.

Fleishman SB and Lesko LM. Delirium and dementia. In Holland J and Rowland J (eds): *Handbook of Psychooncology.* New York, Oxford University Press, 1989.

Grossman SA and Moynihan TA. Neoplastic meningitis. *Neurol Clin* 1991; 9 : 843-56.

Kramer JA. Spinal cord compression in malignancy. *Palliative Med* 1992; 6 : 202-11.

McNamara P *et al.* Use of midazolam in palliative care. *Palliative Med* 1991; 5 : 244-9.

Posner JB. Management of brain metastases. *Rev Neurol* 1992; 148 : 477-87.

Smith MJ *et al.* A critique of instruments and methods to detect, diagnose, and rate delirium. *J Pain Symptom Manage* 1995; 10 : 35-77.

Psychiatric

Billings JA and Block S. Depression. *J Palliative Care* 1995; 11 : 48-54.

Breibart W and Holland JC (eds) : *Psychiatric aspects of symptom management in cancer patients.* Washington DC, American Psychiatric Press, 1993.

Breibart W. Psycho-oncology : depression, anxiety, delirium. *Sem Oncol* 1994; 21 : 754-69.

Holland JC and Rowland JH (eds). *Handbook of Psychooncology. Psychological care of the patient with cancer.* Oxford University Press, 1989.

Endocrine and Metabolic

Harvey HA. The management of hypercalcemia of malignancy. *Support Cancer Care* 1995; 3 : 123-9.

Kovacs CS *et al.* Hypercalcemia of malignancy in the palliative care setting : a treatment strategy. *J Pain Symptom Manage* 1995; 10 : 224-32.

Moertel CG *et al.* The management of patients with advanced carcinoid tumors and islet cell carcinomas. *Ann Int Med* 1994; 120 : 302-9.

Ralston S. Management of cancer-associated hypercalcaemia. *Eur J Palliative Care* 1994; 1 : 170-5.

Constitutional

Bruera E and Higginson I (eds). *Cachexia-anorexia in cancer patients.* Oxford University Press, 1996.

Dunphy K *et al.* Rehydration in palliative and terminal care : if not - why not? *Palliative Med* 1995; 9 : 221-8.

Ellershaw JE *et al.* Dehydration and the dying patient. *J Pain Symptom Manage* 1995; 10 : 192-7.

Levy A. Why flush? *Lancet* 1996; 347 : 73-4.

Piper BF. Fatigue and cancer : inevitable companions? *Support Cancer Care* 1993; 1 : 285-6.

Shaw C. Nutritional aspects of advanced cancer. *Palliative Med* 1992; 6 : 105-10.

Waller A *et al.* The effect of intravenous fluid infusion on blood and urine parameters of hydration and on state of consciousness in terminal cancer patients. *Am J Hosp Palliative Care* 1994; 11 : 22-7.

Index

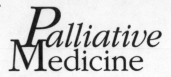